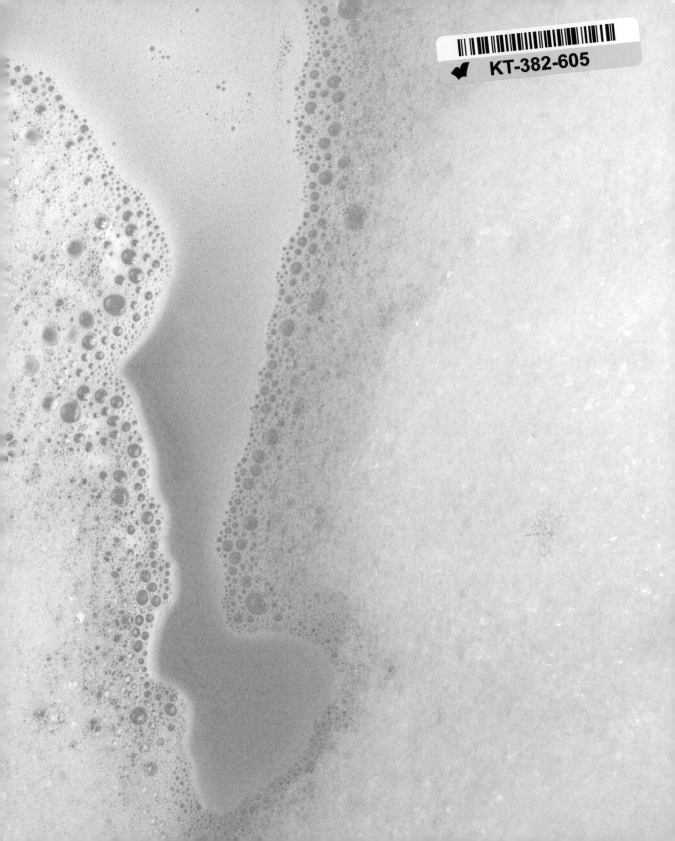

# TOO POSH TO WASH

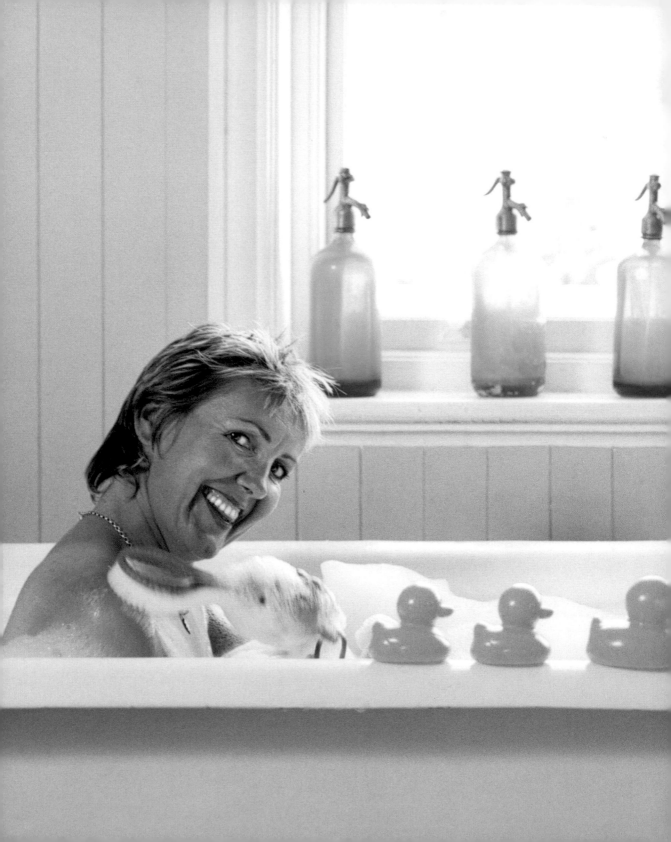

# TOO POSH TO WASH

## KIM WOODBURN AND AGGIE MACKENZIE

MICHAEL JOSEPH

an imprint of PENGUIN BOOKS

Aggie: For my boys, who should know better, and Sorrelle, who always did.

Kim: To Annie Sweetbaum and Debbie Schiesser, my agents from Arlington Enterprises Ltd, and Luigi Bonomi, my literary agent. Without you the book would not have been possible.

MICHAEL JOSEPH
Published by the Penguin Group
Penguin Books Ltd, 80 Strand, London WC2R ORL, England
Penguin Putnam Inc., 375 Hudson Street, New York, New York 10014, USA
Penguin Books Australia Ltd, 250 Camberwell Road, Camberwell, Victoria 3124, Australia
Penguin Books Canada Ltd, 10 Alcorn Avenue, Toronto, Ontario, Canada M4V 3B2
Penguin Books India (P) Ltd, 11 Community Centre,
Panchsheel Park, New Delhi – 110 017, India
Penguin Books (NZ) Ltd, Cnr Rosedale and Airborne Roads,
Albany, Auckland, New Zealand
Penguin Books (South Africa) (Pty) Ltd, 24 Sturdee Avenue,
Rosebank 2196, South Africa

Penguin Books Ltd, Registered Offices: 80 Strand, London WC2R ORL, England

www.penguin.com

First published 2004
1

Text © Fremantle Media Ltd, 2004
Photography © Mark Read, 2004
Design and layout © Michael Joseph, 2004

The moral right of the authors has been asserted

Set in Thesis Sans and New Clarendon
Designed and typeset by Smith & Gilmour, London
Photography: Mark Read
Project Editor: Gillian Haslam
Printed in Great Britain by Butler & Tanner, Frome, Somerset

A CIP catalogue record for this book is available from the British Library

ISBN 0718147693

# Contents

Introduction  6

The bare necessities  16

Bug's life  30

How to wash  38

Bits and pieces  72

Foot and hand notes  108

Home laundry  128

The living environment  160

Clean routines  178

Index  190

Acknowledgements  192

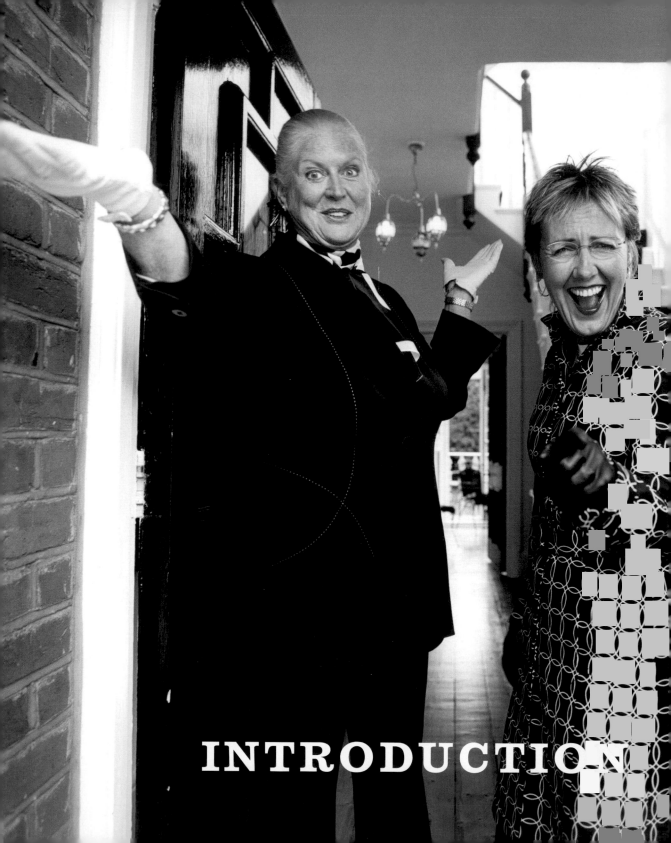

INTRODUCTION

We had a lot of fun sweeping, scrubbing and making Britain's homes sparkle. Oh, what a joy it's been to pull on the rubber gloves and help the nation's mucky pups get the upper hand over their home-grown slime and grime.

But we've met some shockers and stinkers on our travels. And it's not just their homes that honk. At times we've noticed a distinct whiff rising off some people, too. Yes, we're talking smelly armpits, niffy knickers, knock-you-sideways breath, unwashed socks and matted hair. We've been shocked to find how many dirty, unhygienic honkers from all walks of life are living amongst us. Lovely people, but phew, what a stink.

These people don't have any good reason for the sorry state they've got into. They're just soap-dodgers, the poor souls, uninformed about the benefits of cleanliness and the terrible dangers of dirt. So we've decided to sort them out and do everyone – especially their friends and families – a favour.

We've loved sprucing them up, getting into all their little nooks and crannies and scrubbing until they're squeaky clean. But it's not just ingrained dirt, it's their unwashed attitudes. Some of these cheeky monkeys have claimed they're whiffy because they like going 'natural' and don't agree with putting chemicals on their body. We have the answer to that! Soap and water on a daily basis! There is no excuse for stinking the place out.

These soap-dodgers don't realise that there are billions of bugs, bacteria and fungi that thrive on unwashed bodies. These breed and burrow, spread themselves around and cause nasty diseases. It's terrifying for the rest of us. So, assisted in our work by a scientific laboratory, we've donned our white coats and taken swabs from the mucky pups. When that smelly lot see what really goes on under their armpits or between their toes, we hope it frightens them into washing on a daily basis.

We've been shocked by what we've found: teenagers with something approaching trench foot; grown-ups who don't wash their hands after doing a number two, then eat with their fingers. And it doesn't bear thinking about how many men wear the same pants day after day, back to front and inside out so they don't have to wash them.

We've packed these pages with info on personal hygiene and grooming, including the natural, eco-friendly tips we have used in the series, and much, much more. After reading it no-one has any excuse for not being a washed, groomed and sweet-smelling credit to themselves, their friends and family.

So what are you waiting for? Let's get washing!

# All this dirty business has to stop!

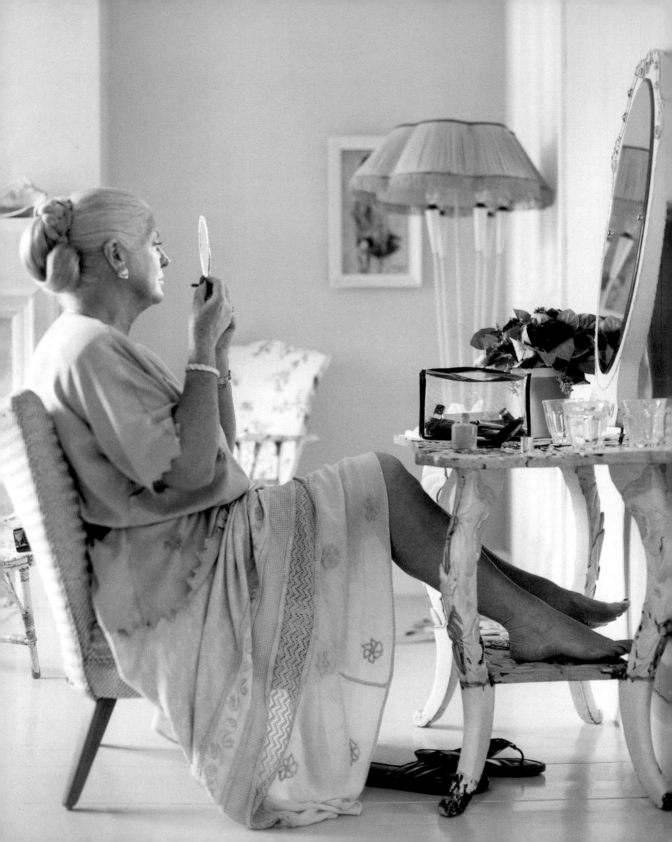

# Kim

Kim has always been keenly interested in beauty and grooming – she trained as a model and worked as a beautician before becoming one half of the 'Nation's Dream Cleaning Team'. As a child, she used to dry rose petals to make perfume, inspired by her glamorous mother's purple bottles of the then fashionable scent, Evening in Paris. 'My tomboy older sister would say, "Ugh, what are you putting that pongy stuff on for?" but I loved it,' Kim says. 'You're born the way you are, and I was born wanting to be girlie and feminine.'

With her soignée but retro blonde hairdo, imposing height and, shall we say, larger than average bust, she certainly stands out from the crowd. 'They call me the Widow Twankey of filth,' exclaims Kim, 'but I've never been one for following beauty fashion. You wear the style that suits you or you look a dope.'

Kim and her husband Peter live in Kent, where he looks after a sheik and his holiday home. Kim loves trying out a myriad of new home beauty treatments. She does her own make-up and hair for telly but treats herself to regular manicures and pedicures. 'I've got shocking eyesight, so I can't do my own toenails. Blimey O'Reilley, with my huge bust, I can't see my feet anyway!'

Kim modestly puts her youthful good looks down to her ability to sleep like the dead. '"Go to bed and look young," I say. I like to lie in and rot.' As she travels the country cleaning up the nation's stinkiest soap-dodgers, she always takes her own emergency grooming kit. Essentials include a white hankie for stains, clean underwear, toothpicks, toothbrush, toothpaste and face wipes. 'You know when you're clean,' Kim says, 'and I like to be clean for as much of the day as I possibly can.'

# Aggie

Aggie was encouraged to pursue rigorous standards of personal hygiene at an early age by her super-clean mum. The highlight of the week was Saturday night, when she and her sisters all got into their weekly bath for a supervised all-over scrub.

You can imagine her excitement at the thought of sorting out the Great British public's personal hygiene on Too Posh To Wash. 'This is right up my street,' she says. 'I just love getting down and dirty and squeezing, prodding, poking and unearthing bits of flotsam and jetsam from the human body.'

She has poked her immaculately polished nails into people's most intimate and stinky places, taking swabs and finding out just what bacteria are lurking there. The results often shock her victims into a regular washing routine. 'It is amazing to me that these people don't wash. They get engrossed in other things – studying or work – and don't notice their stinky smell. Well, enough of that.'

Aggie lives in London with her architect husband Matthew and their sons Rory, 13, and Ewan, 9. Despite her eternal pleadings, the boys still agree to shower only once every other day. Still, Aggie's own personal hygiene routine hasn't changed much since she and Kim shot to fame as the 'Nation's Dream Cleaning Team' two years ago.

At heart, she is a minimalist. 'I like things quick, easy, efficient – it's done with no messing. Then I can get on with the really important things in life.' Like family, baking and tending her allotment.

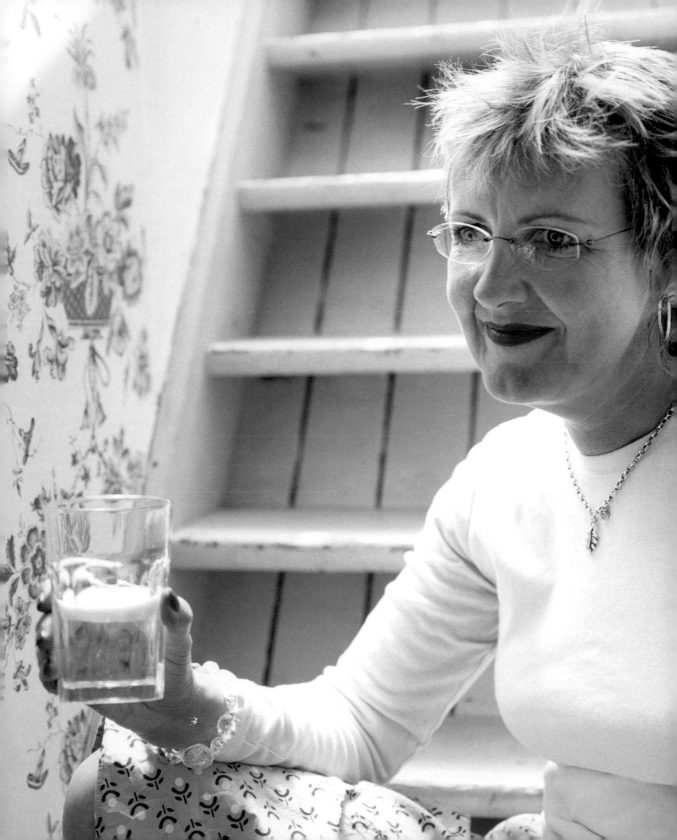

# Are you too posh to wash?

It's unlikely you're as stinky as the hopeless honkers we've had on the show. Still, there might be the odd bit of fluff and stuff in your nooks and crannies that you'd rather we didn't poke our fingers into. You might have some pretty dodgy personal habits that friends and family are too polite to mention.

Are you squeaky clean, or a bit of a stinker? Be truthful, now, this is your chance to come clean!

*Which of the following statements best describes your approach to personal hygiene?*

A  I like to bath or shower every day.
B  I wash regularly, but I don't always have time to make it a daily priority.
C  It's bad for your skin to wash too often. Once every few days is fine.
D  I like my personal aroma – it's what makes me, me.

*How often do you wash your hands after using the toilet?*

A  Every time, with soap and hot water.
B  I always rinse them, but only use soap after a number two.
C  Probably twice a day – that's enough.
D  I don't go in for that soap and water lark.

*Would you ever use someone else's toothbrush?*

A  No, I don't want their bacteria inside my mouth.
B  If I was desperate. I'd rather that than go without brushing my teeth at all.
C  Yes, I don't mind. They're my friends, so why not?
D  I never use one – so it wouldn't apply to me.

*Would you wear the same underpants two days running?*

A  No. I put on a clean pair every morning without fail.
B  I have been known to, if I don't have any clean ones around.
C  Quite often. I turn them inside out so you don't notice.
D  Actually, I can usually go two weeks in the same pants.

*How often do you wash your sheets?*

A  Once a week at least.
B  Once every few weeks – they really don't smell at all.
C  I do it when I can see the dirt.
D  Why waste my time? After all, I only sleep there.

*Do you ever pee in the shower?*

A  No, never, it's unhygienic, repulsive and disgusting.
B  I have done once or twice, rather than getting out of the shower.
C  Quite often. It all goes down the same plughole, doesn't it?
D  Yes, of course. My loo is blocked up something rotten.

*When did you last dust and vacuum
your bedroom?*

**A** This week. I try to keep the dust mite
population down.

**B** I gave it a quick swish a few weeks ago.

**C** It doesn't need it, it's the least dirty room
in the house.

**D** I don't own a vacuum cleaner.

*Your new partner sometimes smells, and
their bedroom is filthy. What would you do?*

**A** Ask them to clean up, or you'll break up.

**B** Leave bars of soap and deodorant around
and hope they get the message.

**C** Say nothing: you're no cleaning maestro
yourself.

**D** We're happy to wallow together.

## Your washing profile

### Mostly As

We're proud of you, dear. You are as bright and
sparkling as a new pin. You take the time to look
and smell lovely, and that is very heartwarming
after all the filthy beggars we've had to deal with
recently. It's a delight to have you on board.

### Mostly Bs

You can scrub up well when you have to,
but there are days when your washing and
grooming routines go to hell in a handbasket.
Smarten yourself up, dear, and stop the
slovenly behaviour. With a little effort you'll
be squeaky clean. You'll feel a whole lot
better and, goodness, so will we.

### Mostly Cs

As if filthy habits and filthier pants are
anything to be proud of! You'll smell rotten
enough when you're in the grave, so why
smell bad when you're alive, for goodness
sake. You need to start scrubbing, before
it's too late and we all pass out.

### Mostly Ds

There should be a law against people like
you. You seriously need to clean up your act!
Read this book from cover to cover, preferably
in the bath, or we'll be round to give you such
a tongue-lashing you'll be sorry you were
ever born.

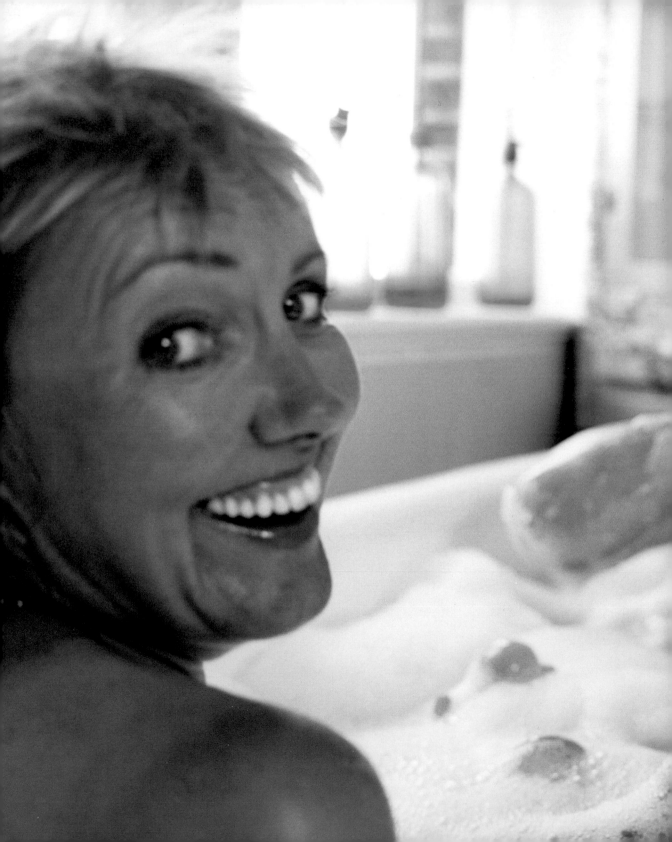

# THE BARE NECESSITIES

# 'I don't wash much, I like my own natural smell …'

We've lost count of the times people repeated this to us in defence of their shoddy hygiene habits. Stinky people believe they smell lovely. They have to, because nobody else does, that's for sure.

Cleanliness is a modern luxury, and don't we all take it for granted! We're so lucky to have every convenience at our fingertips – hot and cold running water, flushing loos, washing machines and vacuum cleaners – that we've forgotten the link between dirt and disease.

# Brief history of man

Dirt kills. Over the ages, millions upon millions of people have died because they couldn't wash their hands in clean water.

Terrible killers such as smallpox, cholera, dysentery, plague and typhoid spread like wildfire in putrid, insanitary conditions. And goodness, were conditions insanitary! In Roman times, public latrines contained a bucket of salt water with a sponge tied onto a stick. After doing their business, people would wipe their pooey bits with the sponge, dunk it back in the salt water and leave it for the next poor sucker who came along. No wonder they died young!

In the olden days, cesspits and water closets had to be cleared out by hand because there were no drains to carry the waste away. Men had to get down into the stinking pits, chuck the bacteria-ridden excrement into carts, then carry it off to throw away in nearby rivers. They often wouldn't bother to wash themselves after.

In the Middle Ages, people had a superstitious fear of water. Even Samuel Pepys believed he caught a cold just by washing his feet. The Black Death, an outbreak of bubonic plague spread by flea-ridden rats, filth and bad sanitation, wiped out one and a half million people – a third of England's population at the time – in just two years.

It's hard to credit now, but flowing drains and fresh, running water only came about in Queen Victoria's reign. Public sanitation became a priority after a string of cholera epidemics claimed thousands of lives. Thereafter, if you were lucky enough to have a water supply, you'd be able to wash your body with a face flannel and a basin of cold water every day if you liked. What a treat!

As people's daily washing habits improved, they started to live longer, happier, less disease-ridden lives. Since the 1870s life expectancy has nearly doubled. You see how good health depends on good hygiene!

The Ancient Greeks had to scrape themselves with an iron tool and rough powder to get the dirt and sweat off. Now we can shower and use soap and deodorants to keep ourselves fresh and clean. There's absolutely no excuse for smelling less than lovely.

## Can you be too clean?

There is a theory that being too clean is bad for us. Some scientists suggest that too much cleanliness is causing a rise in allergies such as asthma, hayfever and atopic dermatitis.

Well, we firmly believe you can never be too clean! Allergies are rising because there's far too much dust around. People who live in stuffy, centrally heated houses provide a perfect breeding ground for dust mites, those nasty little arachnids whose faeces are known to cause allergies. People who don't dust or open their windows to air their rooms unwittingly let mites colonise their beds, and so they breathe in thousands of minuscule allergens every day. No wonder they feel ill.

# too clean?
## phooey to all that!

Of course, some folks are compulsive washers, and they give the rest of us a bad name. Howard Hughes, for instance, a mega-rich American, would use 15 tissues to open his bathroom cabinet, and after visiting the loo would wash his hands four times using four different bars of soap. That, dear, is bonkers! You don't need to get obsessive about personal hygiene. Regular hand washing and sluicing the body daily with hot water and soap are good enough.

# Kim and Aggie's essential grooming kit

Look around the shelves of any chemist and you'll see a breathtaking array of grooming and beauty products. They promise wonders and are so temptingly packaged that it's hard to navigate your way around the shelves without spending a fortune. Some products are excellent, but you don't need to buy five different ones for five different areas of the body – that's hardly economical. Still, every person needs some basic grooming products to suit their skin, hair and lifestyle. Even the stinky so-and-sos we visited had soap and shampoo, they just didn't use them on a regular basis!

# Aggie

I like a streamlined bathroom cabinet – I can't be doing with ten different products when just one will suffice. I don't worry too much about what soap and shampoo I use but I am fussy about my tweezers and nail scissors – I've had both for 20 years. This is the essential kit I swear by.

## Grooming essentials

### Tweezers

I love tweezing, but I've never got around to those posh tweezers. I've got a pair in my Swiss Army knife, which I always carry with me. At home I have ones with flat, thin ends which makes the tweaking easier. For handiness in the bathroom, I always put my tweezers over the edge of the tooth mug. So when I look in the mirror and see a stray hair I don't take my eyes off it for a second. I reach over for the tweezers and swipe – it's out!

### Toothbrush

I don't use an electric one. I know they're meant to be better but I never got on with them. I like doing the hand movement regime myself: up and down, in and out, into all those wee nooks and crannies – two minutes at least. I'm probably too hard on the gums but rather that than a dirty mouth.

### Razor

I once had my underarms waxed. It was like giving birth to oversized twins and I've never been brave enough to do it again. Now I use one of those lady's razors to do my underarms and bikini area. I get into such trouble if I ever use my husband's blade – he always knows.

### Men's razors

I like a man who wet shaves. I think it's very manly and you get a closer shave too. I bought my husband a pure bristle shaving brush for Christmas and he uses the solid soap to get a lovely lather up.

### Electric exfoliator

I can't be doing with stubble on my legs, so I use one of those electric tweezers which plucks the hairs out at the roots. If I don't have time for that, I'd rather get a leg wax than shave – it's painful but I enjoy it in a funny way.

### Hairbrush and comb

I don't actually use a brush or comb myself. My hair is so short I just wash it every day then muss it up. But for the rest of the family I like those lovely, black, shiny brushes and a good, solid, tortoiseshell comb, wide-toothed so you're not tearing your hair out.

### Towels

Buy white only, so you can see if they're getting skanky. I love a rough towel, not those soft fluffy ones. I like a bit of abrasion on the skin, it's my tough Scottish upbringing. With a hard towel you get the blood going and feel zingy afterwards.

### Nail scissors

I cut the nails of everyone in the house – I even do my husband's toenails. I use the nail scissors I've had for 20 years, the little dinky ones with a straight edge which I got in a DIY shop. They get right down into the cheesy bits in the corners, and it's so satisfying when it comes out in one chunk. I like the feeling of cutting off the nail in a long bit too – like peeling an orange in one go.

'I like a shower – I think they're more hygienic. In a bath you're sitting in all your muck and when you stand up there's scum all over your body. But there are times when a bath can be just the ticket. When my feet are aching and I feel filthy, I can't get into the bath fast enough.'

# Grooming goo

### Soap

I like translucent soap, though it does erode very quickly. It's got that lovely, sharp, clean smell which reminds me of Saturday nights as a kid when I and my sisters had a soak in the big bath. I don't like shower gel – just one more thing to worry about. I just use a bar of soap, and it goes all over. It's cheaper and it doesn't dry your skin out.

### Hair gel

I slick this on every day. Choose one which suits your hair type with the strength of hold you want.

### Toothpaste

I buy whatever's on special offer – everyone loves a bargain. My favourite is a pump action one. I know they're wasteful, but they're clean. With tubes you get too much gummy paste around the head of the nozzle. And then someone leaves the top off the tube and the germs get in.

### Deodorant

I always use a roll on, never a spray. A deodorant has to be odourless, so it doesn't interfere with my perfume.

### Shampoo

Any one will do so long as it smells herby, like rosemary or thyme. I can't see much difference between cheap and expensive shampoos, so why waste your money?

### Conditioner

I use it every day because I've got colour in my hair. Almost any will do. I just put a blob on, leave for minute while I wash the rest of my body, then rinse out thoroughly.

### Dental floss

I don't use dental floss often enough – I always seem to forget before bed. Anyway, I prefer the sticks because you can poke away at all that smelly, minging stuff between your teeth and it gives your gums a good massage at the same time.

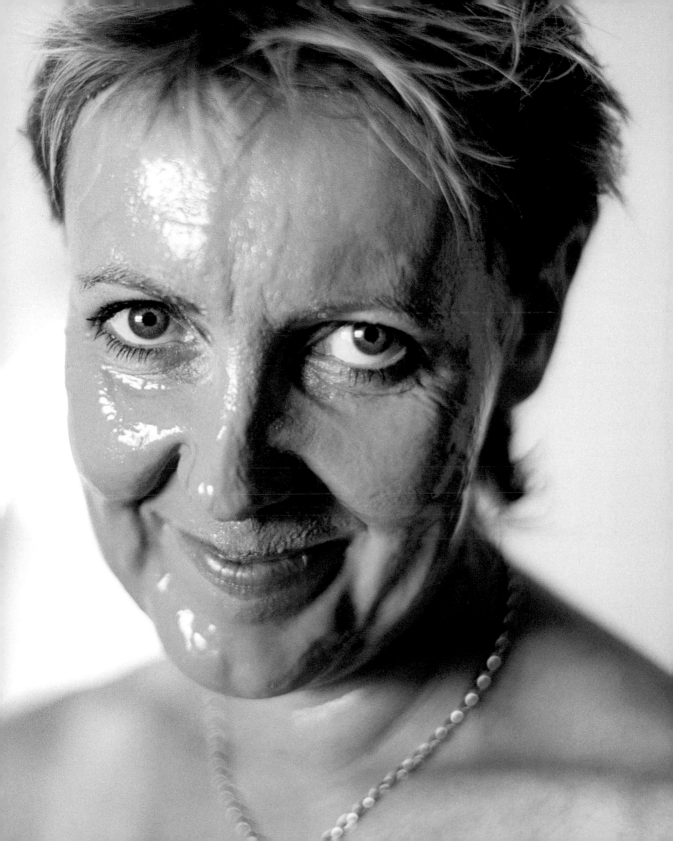

# Kim

I like to be feminine. I set out to look nice, and these are the tried and tested grooming tools and products I've used over the years, although I do love trying out new nail varnishes and make-up. I moisturise my face and neck everyday, but if a product promises to get rid of the wrinkles, it's utter rubbish. You can soften wrinkles, but only surgery will take them away.

## Grooming essentials

### Hairbrush and comb

I use a bristle hairbrush and I have two plastic combs – one very wide-toothed comb for when hair is wet, and one close-toothed tail comb. My hair is long and I tear the gibbons out of it if I use a normal comb when it's wet. The tail comb smoothes down the front of my hair so it's spot on before I lacquer it.

### Toothbrush

The dentist will kill me for saying this, but I love nothing better than a soft, frayed, old toothbrush. It wiggles in and out of all the crevices in the mouth and captures everything. Some people's toothbrushes make you want to vomit. There's fried egg and everything in there! But I keep mine spotless. Once a week I soak it in washing-up liquid, then rinse in warm water, bang it on a towel and it's clean.

### Nailbrush

I like a soft nailbrush. Hard ones are all right for engine drivers but I don't want them, thank you. Once a day I run the nailbrush over the toilet soap, slip it under my nails and give them a good clean. It's done in two seconds. I always rinse it out, then bang it on the side of the sink. You can clean behind your nails with wooden cocktail sticks, too, but it takes ages.

### Pumice stone

Essential! You see women in sandals with grey, cracked heels – all they need to do is get the pumice stone out. At the very first sign of dry skin I pummy around the back of my heels and big toes in the bath, then slather on the cream and put a pair of old socks on top. An hour later your feet are lovely and soft.

**Tweezers**

I'm not fussy about my tweezers. I like small ones and, as long as the two nibs meet very well in the middle, I can cope.

**Emery boards**

I don't use clippers or scissors. I've got long nails, and if you cut them you can crack them in the middle. Instead, I use emery boards. Fine or thick. I never use a metal file on my nails. I file the length down with the rough side, then shape with the smooth side to finish them off.

**Towels**

It's got to be white cotton – I like knowing exactly where my dirt is. There's nothing wrong with black and red towels, except the dye comes out of them and you can't wash them with anything else. I change my towels nearly every day, too.

**Face flannel**

I use one every day. White or maybe pale pink or blue for a change. I wash it every day. I soak it with some toilet soap or biological washing powder for half an hour, then rinse and throw it back on the bath rack.

**Dental floss**

It's stunning stuff, but I can't get into a habit with it. I use wooden cocktail sticks instead to get between my teeth. If I'm out in a restaurant it makes me sick to see the person opposite me sucking and picking at their teeth. Instead, I put my toothpick in my bag, pop to the loo and have a quiet dig around and pick any food out.

**Razor**

I wet shave under my arms every day, and if anything grows, whoosh, it's gone. I use a lady's razor, but get one that suits your own hair growth, whether it's coarse or fine.

'I have a bubble bath every single day. I think women need to sit their nether regions in the bath, it's the way we're made. I feel fresh after a bath, it's very feminine. I always finish off with a quick shower to get rid of the soap.'

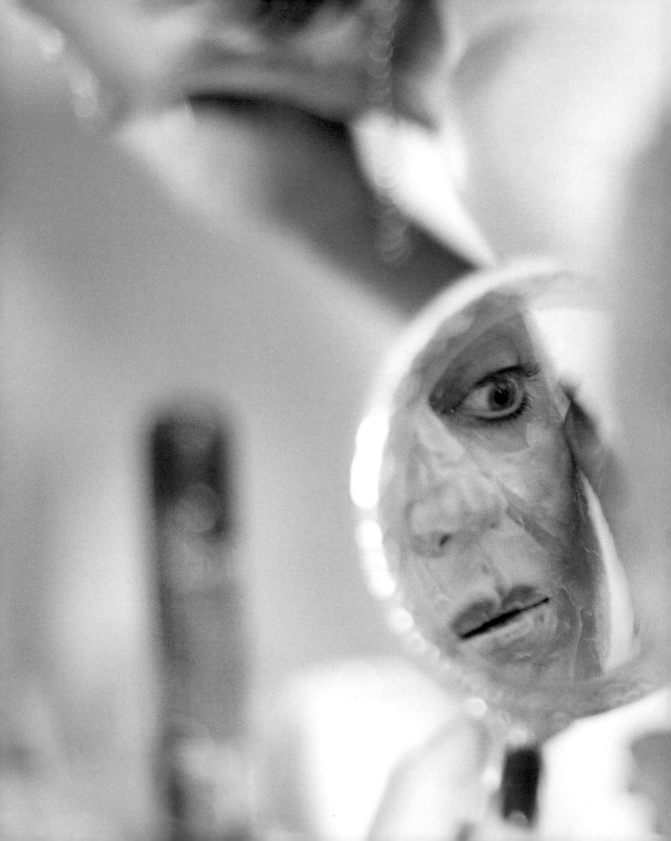

# Grooming goo

### Bubble bath
Ooh, I love it. I have a bath every day and use a peach bubble bath. It's very creamy and good for dry skin. Afterwards, I rinse off in the shower to get rid of any soapy residue that could give you the itches.

### Soap
I use a pretty soap with a light musk fragrance. It's not sweet or sickly, but it has a nice feminine smell.

### Deodorant
I like a roll-on antiperspirant. One of those moist ones, not the thick, powdery ones that leave a white sticky mess all over your clothes. They are atrocious – whoever invented them ought to be shot.

### Moisturiser and night cream
I put moisturiser on every morning before I do my make-up – it flows on better. At night, if my skin feels dry, I'll put the same cream on half an hour before going to bed to give it time to absorb. If you put it on any later, the pillow will be like a greaseball.

### Toothpaste and whitener
I brush my teeth three times a day. I clean first with pure white, mint toothpaste – I don't like a gel. Then I use a special whitener afterwards. You just brush it on and ooh, it makes a difference. You can see it right away.

### Shampoo
With blondes it's very hard to get a shine on your hair. The right shampoo can help but you have to find it first. I use one for dry hair, but look at the hair you've got. None of them work miracles, so buy small sizes until you establish one that's good for you.

### Conditioner
If you use lots of hairspray, you need conditioner. I wash my hair every other day and always use a great deal of conditioner. If I'm in for the evening, I'll slather it on, wrap my hair in a warm towel and potter round with it on for a couple of hours. It works wonders.

### Hairspray
I use it every day – my hair is like a crash helmet when I'm filming. Even if you use a hard hold hairspray, you want to get it all out at the end of the day. I always use one that brushes out easily.

### Talcum powder
I love my talc. I like to pat it around my body every morning after my bath. It keeps you dry and smells lovely and feminine.

### Hand cream
Use a cheap one, dear, and don't break the bank. I find ordinary ones or those for babies work best. They're not heavily perfumed and you can slather them up your arms, too.

# BUG'S
# LIFE

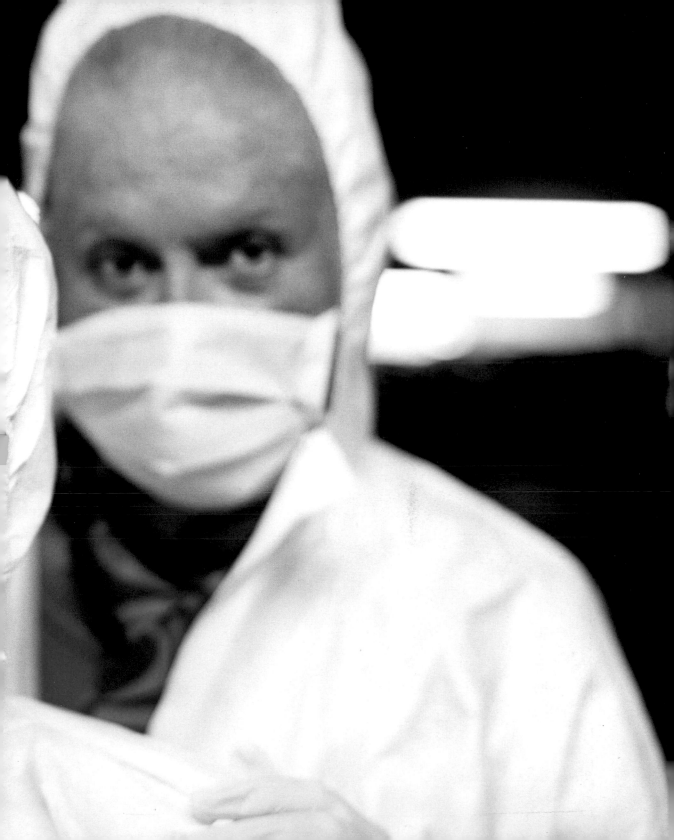

We were horrified by the beasties and bacteria we found lingering on some members of the Great British public. We had to put on our decontamination suits, masks, gloves and wellies just to get near these bug-infested blighters. Poor old Ags was poking and prodding in all their bodily cavities, searching out the grungy places where bacteria hide. Isn't she the brave one!

Using our dirt detective bags and swabs, we took samples from these stinkers. The results were shocking! Billions of dangerous bacteria were growing willy-nilly on the bodies of the great unwashed. Some bugs are good for us, so the experts say, but goodness, these were getting wildly out of hand.

There were plenty of pests feeding off the skin and detritus of filth offenders. They spread germs and diseases which can cause food poisoning, allergies and other nasty illnesses. Who wants to be a 24-hour larder for bugs and insects?

# Wee crawling beasties

## Bed bugs

Did you hear that these dreadful creatures are making a comeback? They're a real horror story. They come out at night, usually just before dawn, to feed on the blood of sleeping innocents. In the olden days, people used to creep into their bedrooms, pull back the covers and bash at the bed with a bar of soap to kill as many as they could.

Oh they're clever little blighters, though. They can exist for months without a meal, and they migrate around in luggage, second-hand furniture and old mattresses.

Bed bugs' mouths are designed to pierce and suck and they can take in up to four times their body weight in blood.

Although they don't carry diseases, their saliva causes irritation and a hard, white swelling to form.

You can tell you've got bed bugs if you wake up with itchy spots in the morning and there are small speckles of red blood (yours) and brown excreta (theirs) over your sheets.

Never buy old mattresses, and check over second-hand furniture thoroughly before bringing it into the house.

If you suspect an infestation, call in your local council pest control.

**APPLIANCE OF SCIENCE**
Adult bed bugs live for nine to 18 months, and females lay up to three eggs a day. They don't need food to survive: they can live from four months to a year without consuming a single drop of blood.

# Scabies

An itch mite which makes its home on your skin, usually on the hands, wrists, feet, armpits, genitals and around the navel. Having scabies is like being colonised by the living dead. The females burrow tiny passageways into the skin which they fill up with eggs – then they die. When the eggs hatch a few weeks later, the allergic rashes and itching start with a vengeance. You'll be scratching day and night, and skin can quickly get infected.

Scabies mites are so small you can't see them, but they are easily transferred from one person to another.

Left untreated, scabies can lead to eczema and other chronic skin conditions. If sites get infected, blood poisoning can result.

Scabies can spread via bed linen, shared clothing, or hand-to-hand contact. About 300 million people in the world suffer from scabies at any one time.

Topical treatments kill scabies mites – see your GP if you suspect you have them.

**APPLIANCE OF SCIENCE**
Most bacteria, fungi and viruses like a nice, moist environment so thrive in damp places like toilets. But germs can also live for several hours on:
* Magazines and books
* Door handles
* Taps
* Toilet handles
* Pool cues
* Light switches
* Telephones
* Clothes
* Furniture
* Your own and other people's hands

'Cleanliness becomes more important when godliness is unlikely.' P J O'Rourke

# Fungi

It's not nice to think you're lunch for millions of bacteria. But we haven't yet mentioned the nasty growths and fungi that attach themselves to unwashed bodies at the drop of a hat. Common irritations like jock itch, athlete's foot, barber's itch, dandruff, thrush and ringworm are all caused by fungal infection. And you smell these ones before you see them!

Like pollen and dust mites, fungi also cause allergies in the respiratory tract. At various times of the year, there are more fungal spores in the air than pollen grains.

Fungi are invisible parasites that munch away at skin whenever they get the opportunity. You can pick them up all over the place – at swimming pools, from rugs, from shared towels – and once you've got them, they can live almost indefinitely in the skin.

Gives you something to chew on, doesn't it?

# Head lice

These beasties don't care what condition your hair is in, they just want a good meal. Young schoolchildren are always picking them up, and budget long-haul travellers can come back with a dose of Delhi belly and hair crawling with head lice and baby nits. Cut hair short before you go.

These bloodsuckers are only tiny but they can crawl like the blazes when they need to. They're mostly found around the ears and at the back of the neck, where it's nice and warm, and where they lay their eggs.

By tramping around all over your head, piercing and sucking as they go, they cause an itchy irritation and inflammation which can drive you mad.

Head lice are transferred by head-to-head contact, and by sharing hats, scarves, brushes and combs.

To treat: use a proprietary nit lotion recommended by your pharmacist and comb through with a fine-toothed nit comb every few days.

When wet, head lice are unable to move, so are easier to comb out.

APPLIANCE OF SCIENCE
* Female head lice lay from three to 10 eggs a day, which take a week to hatch. They then need a bloody meal from your scalp within 24 hours.
* Head lice can move fast: about 23cm (9 inches) in 60 seconds.
* Body lice are associated with diseases such as typhus, trench fever and relapsing fever.
* In dirty, overcrowded conditions these diseases can be fatal.

# Bacteria

We don't like to think of it but there are millions of bacteria that exist in and on us. Mostly we aren't aware of them and they don't harm us, especially when we keep clean and practise good hand washing and food hygiene routines. But sometimes these little blighters can make us ill. Here are a few of the worst offenders.

### Staphylococcus aureus

This bug is everywhere, and it can be a nasty one. Most of us carry it around on our skin and in our noses. So don't go picking your snozzle, or you can get it on your fingers and infect yourself through a cut or graze. It can be sneezed out, too, and spread itself in droplets of mucus.

On the skin, staph can cause boils, pimples, carbuncles, rashes and impetigo, but when it gets inside the body, all hell breaks loose. It can cause food poisoning, pneumonia, and serious bone and blood infections. It can even mutate into that antibiotic-resistant MRSA superbug that some unlucky people catch in hospitals.

In one sneeze you produce up to 20,000 droplets of saliva and mucus, many containing bacteria and viruses. Half of all food poisoning cases are caused by people not washing their hands.

### E. coli

This bug lives in vast numbers in our gut and for the most part helps keep us healthy. But there is a nasty strain called *E. coli 0157*. You can pick it up from faeces or from touching raw meat.

Just 10 of these microscopic bugs can cause illness, with painful tummy cramps, internal bleeding and bloody diarrhoea. Healthy people can shake off the bug, but in very young children and old folk it can be a rampant killer.

One whiffy fellow we had the pleasure of meeting had 64 million bacteria on his hands – including *E. coli* – proof that he had not been washing his hands after using the loo.

### Pseudomonas and Serretia

These bugs are found in water and soil and can cause nasty ear and eye infections. They love damp spots and often live in Jacuzzis, swimming pools, spas, hot tubs – and even in bottled water. These opportunistic little devils can easily infect your mascara wand or contact lens case. And if you have a scratch on the surface of your eye – as contact lens wearers often do – they can quickly colonise your eye, causing loss of vision and, in extreme cases, blindness.

### Listeria and Salmonella

These are present is some foodstuffs, can cause nasty stomach upsets and diarrhoea, and can even be fatal in vulnerable people. Listeria still breeds in cold temperatures and can survive in the fridge – luckily you need to ingest a lot before you get ill. Good food hygiene and hand washing practices stop them spreading.

### Propionibacterium acnes

This bug lives on and in the skin. When pores get blocked due to the overproduction of sebum (oil in the skin), it bubbles away below skin level. The result is infection and inflammation – which erupts in a big pus-filled spot. In no time this can develop into inflammatory acne, where pus-filled cysts rupture beneath the skin's surface, spreading the infection. Keeping the surface of skin clean is half the battle.

**APPLIANCE OF SCIENCE**
Parasites outnumber us! There are around 10 to the power of 14 (100,000,000,000,000) bacterial, fungal, viral and parasitic cells in our bodies, compared to just 10 to the power of 13 (10,000,000,000,000) human cells.

# HOW TO WASH

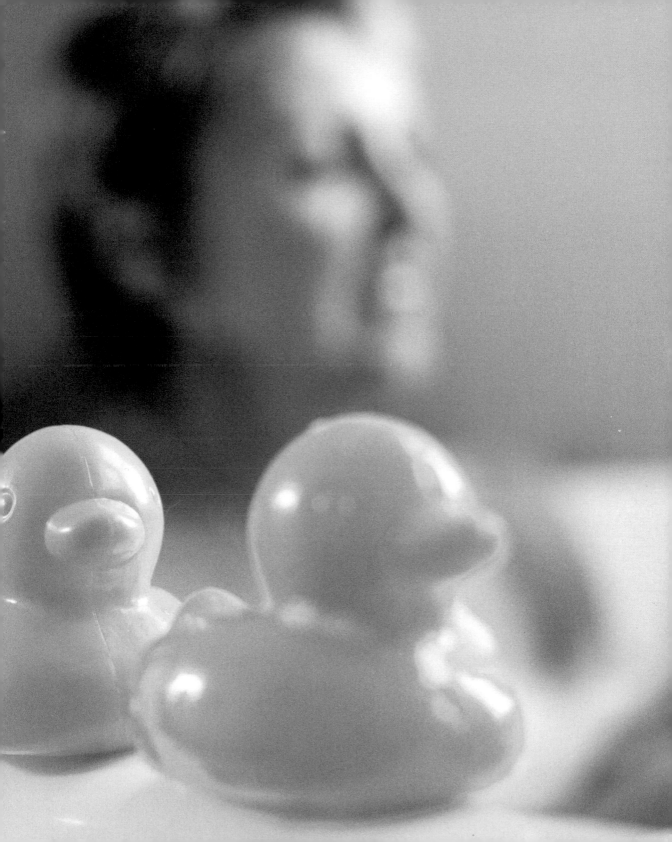

We all sweat a bit but some seem to sweat buckets. And doesn't it pong? On our travels we met some self-confessed stinkers who were proud to admit that their bodies hadn't been near water for weeks. They've got grime behind their ears, dried brine encrusting their armpits and their fetid feet give off a foul stench. They wonder why people cross the street to avoid them!

And it's not just their offensive pong – though that's bad enough. No, these filth offenders also spread their muck around, passing on their deadly biohazards to innocent bystanders. They need to clean up their act with a good daily scrub from top to bottom. A hot, soapy shower sloughs off millions of dead skin cells, parasites and disease-producing micro-organisms – and does us all a favour by getting rid of their nasty niff!

# To BO or not to BO?

There's no excuse for smelling bad, though we've heard a few. We've
lost count of the number of men and women who are proud not to wash.
They've told us that their partners don't mind the smell at all, and they
won't scrub up in case they lose the powerful sexual allure of their
pheromones. Well, pheromones, smellomones, we say. Give us a lovely,
clean body any day.

## Why you need to wash

Dogs regulate their body temperature
by panting, humans do it by perspiring.
There are about three million sweat
glands on the body – just think what
a stink that can cause!

That real peg-on-your-nose pong
comes when a person doesn't wash
the sweat and bacteria off their body
regularly. If they wear the same smelly
clothes day after day, they set up a
sniff cycle that has the rest of us
running for cover.

Most of the stench is caused by the
bacteria feeding on the sweat produced
in the groin and underarm areas.

According to our microbiologist Derren
Ready, regular washing reduces the
number of skin parasites and disease-
producing micro-organisms that can
be transmitted from one person to
another. It also removes body secretions
such as sweat and sebum, as well as the
micro-organisms that feed on them
to produce body odour.

**APPLIANCE OF SCIENCE**
Illnesses spread by dirty
hands include amoebic
dystentery, conjunctivitis,
cholera, gastro-enteritis
from *E. coli* and salmonella,
hepatitis A and E, herpes,
impetigo and typhoid fever.
Many of these are killers!

# What makes us sweat most?

- Hot weather: most people lose between a half to a litre of sweat a day, but in very hot weather we can lose that much in an hour.

- Exercise – so wash it off afterwards!

- Being overweight.

- Anxiety.

- Hot flushes – many women sweat more when they're going through the menopause.

- Drinking alcohol can bring on a hot flush.

- Some foods – garlic, onions and spicy meals like curries.

- Some infections and diseases – for example an overactive thyroid gland.

# It's a crime against hygiene.

**APPLIANCE OF SCIENCE**
There are 60 sweat glands per square centimetre on our backs, and 600 per square centimetre on the soles of our feet. About one per cent of the population sweat excessively – this is called hyperhidrosis and may be genetic.

# How to wash

We've been fortunate to meet some lovely folk along the way, but my goodness some of them were pongy. Lucky that we brought along our own decontamination shower to blast the bacteria off. This is the shower used by troops involved in chemical warfare and it does the business. There's a lovely shooting jet of hot, hot water and you get a good lather up in a minute.

   Mind you, we had to scrub it down well after these deadly odour offenders had done with it. The walls and floor were covered with grime, hair and soapy sludge. It wasn't just weeks, but months some of them had gone without soap and water! There's no excuse for letting yourself get that dirty, it's a crime against hygiene. Our daily five-minute washing routine is all you need to sort yourself out.

# The five-minute boil wash

Sounds nasty, doesn't it? A boil wash might be overheating it a bit, but you do need hot water (but not too hot or it will dry out the natural oils in the skin) and plenty of it to cut through the grease and grime and get yourself clean. We like those electric showers, where you can switch on, jump in, and have a good amount of hot water day or night, whenever you fancy.

**1** Firstly, do the face. Soap can be very drying on the delicate skin here, so we like to wipe with cleanser and splash all over with water instead.

**2** Then give yourself a pre-wash – stand under the water and rub yourself all over to make sure you're thoroughly wet and your skin is zinging. If you want to wash your hair, use a small blob of shampoo, then leave on any conditioner while you wash the rest of your body.

**3** Next, grab the soap and lather under your arms – a good 10 seconds each side, please, and no slacking! Then rub soap and water over your shoulders, neck and arms, and down your sides and back. Use a back scrubber if you can't reach any tricky bits. The soap removes excess oils and prevents the build-up of blocked pores and blackheads.

**4** Then the chest. Men need to lather up well and ladies need to pay particular attention to the cleavage area, which can get hot and sticky in warm weather.

**5** Down to the tummy button, which rarely gets a good clean, so sluice around in there for a bit. Then on to the nether regions, don't stint.

**6** Go down the legs, paying particular attention to the backs of the knees which often get neglected. Then the feet: hold on to the side of the bath, then lift, lather, and rinse off immediately to stop yourself slipping. Make sure you get right between the toes and round the back of your heels where all the dead skin harbours nasty bacteria.

**7** Then it's rinse, rinse, rinse. Take the shower off the hook if you can and point it at your various bits to make sure you're clean and soap-free all over.

**8** There – doesn't that feel better already! And it only took five minutes.

**APPLIANCE OF SCIENCE**
Every day we shed around 500 million skin scales and 10 million of these will carry bacteria and fungi. Skin can never be 100 per cent clean, as it constantly produces sebum and sweat.

# Exfoliate, exfoliate, exfoliate

Skin likes a good rub, much like a pet dog. To get rid of rough
old skin, try an all-over scrub in the shower with oatmeal. Oats
are hypoallergenic, and soften and soothe itchy, dry skin. Mix some
ground oatmeal with water or natural yoghurt to a paste. Rub
on to skin in a gentle circular motion, paying particular attention
to rough areas around the knees and elbows. Rinse well.

**STAR TIP**
Sea salt and olive oil
makes a wonderful body
scrub for the shower.
It's a natural and
cleansing exfoliant.

# The torso sluice

In the olden days, most people didn't have a bathroom with running hot and cold in the house. Goodness no. It's hard to imagine what things were like then when these days you can't turn round in a house without bumping into another en suite bathroom.

Still, mothers were very strict about cleanliness. Every morning, we'd have to wash our hands and face, and every evening we'd do the works – hands, face, neck, underarms and then the bits down there – with a flannel and tin basin in front of the fire. No excuses.

Older folks often still give themselves a daily once-over and if you're ever somewhere where you can't get to a shower or bath, it's your best alternative. We've called our five minute non-biological freshen-up the Torso Sluice. Here's how you do it.

1. Get a basin of hot water, soap and a clean flannel.

2. Start at the cleanest end first – the top. You don't want muck floating around in the bowl while you're washing the rest of you. Wash your face, neck and behind your ears with the wet flannel and just a smidgeon of soap. Rinse.

3. On to the underarms. Lather up the soap on the flannel, then rub around the whole armpit area. Rinse. Give yourself a sniff there to check all is well. If not, wash and rinse again.

4. Now for the nether regions. You need lots of soap here to get rid of any lurking bacteria. Get a nice lather up, give a good scrub, then rinse well.

5. Dry yourself all over, starting at the face.

6. Just look at all the muck and dander in that bowl! Chuck the lot down the sink and wash your flannel straight away. Perfect!

## Face flannels

It's true, they're just one more thing to launder. They get dirty quickly but they are useful, too. We like them for washing the body, for spot cleaning clothes, and Aggie's boys use them to get shampoo out of their eyes when they're washing their hair – it's easier than grabbing a towel. But we use white ones so we can see the grime, and they get washed every day!

# Bathing beauties

Showers get you tingling, dear, but sometimes there's nothing better than the luxury of a good soak to ease the muscles and soothe the mind. Plain water is lovely, but add bubble bath or essential oils to suit your mood: lavender to soothe, rosemary or chamomile for tired muscles, bergamot or lime to lift the spirits. A bath is marvellous for sending you off to the land of nod, too. Dry off well and half an hour later you'll be tucked up and snoozing.

# Botanical bathing tips

**To invigorate skin and stimulate the circulation**
Grate some fresh ginger and tie in an old pop-sock or stocking. Place under the running water while you run the bath.

**To stop itchiness**
A glass of apple cider vinegar in the bath works a treat. Or try one of the emollient bath oils containing liquid paraffin – they cleanse skin, too, so are good for children who don't like using soap. (Ask at the pharmacy counter for the big bargain bottles. They are the same price for nearly twice the amount.)

**To moisturise skin**
Take the skins of four or five lemons or limes and tie them into the foot of a stocking or pop-sock. Place this in the bath. In a few minutes there will be a wonderfully fresh aroma. The citrus oils moisturise skin beautifully. As an alternative, use orange peel.

**For smooth skin**
Add a couple of handfuls of Epsom salts (from a pharmacy) to the bath water.

**To exfoliate skin**
Try a milk bath. The lactic acid in milk is a mild exfoliant. Use powdered milk, not liquid, but don't sprinkle it straight into the bath. Instead, put a cup of powdered milk with some water in a jar and shake well until no lumps are left. Pour into your bath and soak. This removes dead skin cells and leaves you silky smooth.

**To make a bath mitt**
Don't throw out mismatched white cotton socks – they are wonderful as an exfoliant bath mitt. Turn them inside out to the nubbly, abrasive side, put your hand in and rub all over.

**To make a body scrubber**
Save up your old slivers of soap and put them into an old white cotton sock, as above. Tie the sock with a bit of ribbon and you have the perfect soapy scrubber.

# Hands

Oh, the grot we've seen on people's hands, it's been shocking! One soap-dodger's grubby mitts didn't touch water for weeks! It makes you shudder to think of the nasty, infectious bugs he was carrying around with him. There were 64 million bacteria on this king of ming's hands! Lovely lad, mind, but he didn't have a clue that he was a toxic biohazard, spreading germs around to all and sundry.

**APPLIANCE OF SCIENCE**
90 per cent of germs on the hands are found under the nails. The number of bacteria can double in 20 minutes. After one day without hand washing, a single bacterium can multiply 2 billion, trillion times. These bugs can cause diarrhoea, fever and other nasty illnesses.

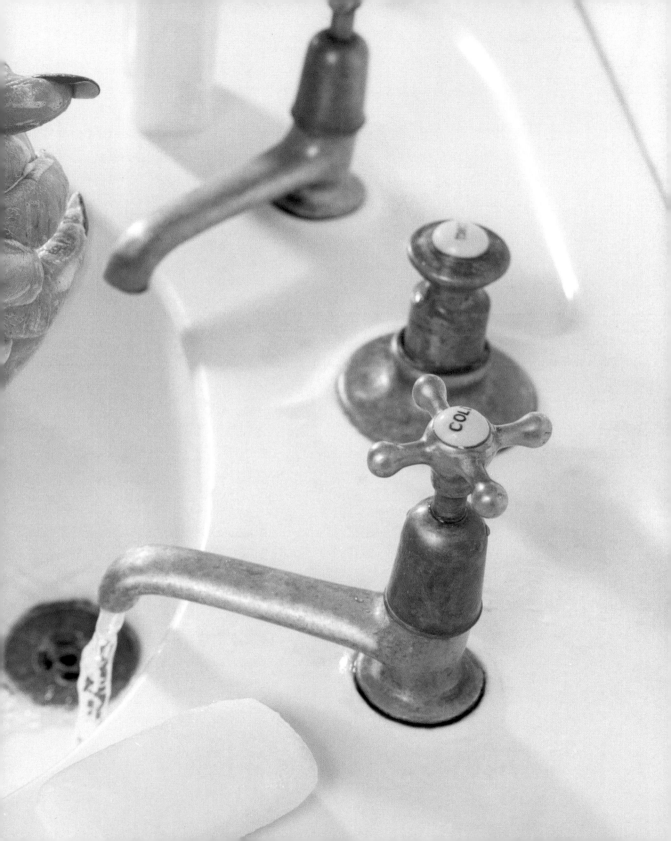

# When to wash your hands

Half of all food poisoning cases come from people not washing their hands. Germs can live on the hands for several hours and spread to anything you touch, from food to door handles to pool cues. This is called faecal-oral transmission and can make you, your family and anyone you come into contact with ill with diarrhoea, cramping, abdominal pain and fever. But it's easy to prevent if you wash your hands:

- After you go to the loo

- Before preparing food or eating

- After changing a baby's nappy

- After emptying rubbish bins

- After handling any raw meat, which can carry salmonella and campylobacter bugs

- After touching pets and animals

- After gardening

**APPLIANCE OF SCIENCE**
Regular hand-washers visit the GP 25 per cent fewer times and use 86 per cent less medication than non-regular hand-washers. Schoolchildren who were taught to wash their hands properly had a 25 per cent reduction in sick days taken off school due to gastrointestinal and respiratory illnesses. When a group of university students improved their hand hygiene, they had significantly fewer illnesses and 43 per cent fewer days off sick.

# The best way to wash your hands

Rinsing your hands under the cold water tap does not count as proper hand washing by a long chalk! Instead try our hand washing recipe. It looks complicated but it soon becomes second nature, we can assure you.

Use warm water and soap – bar or liquid is fine.

Work up a good lather on the palms of your hands.

Work the lather between each finger and on to the backs of hands and rub well. The friction dislodges microbes.

Don't neglect the fingertips – more bacteria live under the nails than anywhere else on the hands.

If you're right handed, you probably wash your left hand more thoroughly, and vice versa. Make sure both hands get a proper going over.

Wash around thumbs well – most of us concentrate on the palms and fingers.

Wash for about 15 to 20 seconds in total.

Rinse with clean, running water.

Drying hands thoroughly on a clean, dry, towel or paper towel will further reduce the number of micro-organisms.

If the skin on your hands gets dry, use a hand cream containing a high percentage of glycerin to prevent soreness and chapping.

STAR TIPS
* Once a day, take off all your jewellery when you wash your hands. Millions of germs hide under rings, bracelets and watches.
* If using a bar of soap, store it in a soap dish with a draining hole so it can dry out.
* If using hand cream, buy a pump dispenser or tube rather than dipping your finger into a jar. This prevents hand creams becoming laden with bacteria.

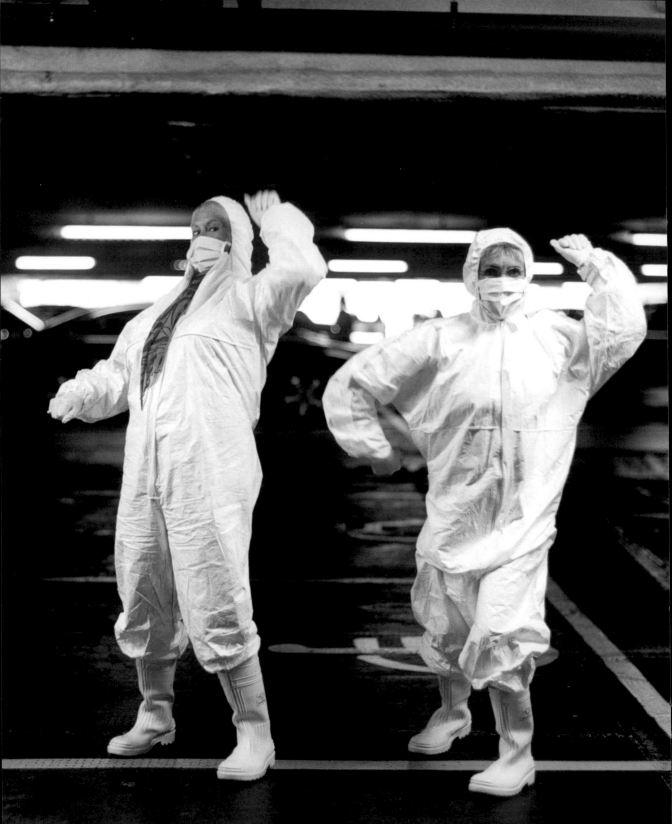

# Public loos

Aren't there some nasty public loos out there? Filthy floors, broken toilet seats, and years of accumulated stains. And the honk! When was the last time these places got a good scrubbing?

In some toilets you've as much chance of spotting loo paper as finding a snowball in hell. Then you find there's only cold water, a cracked bit of dried-up soap and a honking old towel that hasn't been washed since the Crimean War. Your hands are dirtier when you walk out than when you went in.

## How to use a public loo

Before you go in to a cubicle, check there's enough loo paper there for your needs.

However murky it looks, we'd rather have the loo seat down than up – at least then you don't have to see the full stained horror of the porcelain pan. If you have to pull the seat down, use a fingertip or a bit of loo roll so that you hardly touch it.

Wipe the seat with loo roll or a wet wipe if it looks mucky. Some people hover over it rather than sit, but we only do that if it's really nasty.

It's as well to assume the previous person has not washed their hands before touching the toilet handle – how could they, unless there's a basin in the loo? Flush the toilet, pushing the handle with the side of the hand only.

Afterwards, wash hands well with hot soapy water. Use a paper towel to turn off the tap – germs such as E. coli, which are found in faeces, can live on taps for several hours. Kim always carries wet wipes in her handbag in case there's no way of washing her hands.

Dry hands with a paper towel or a roller towel. Dryers can blow bacteria from the loo around the room and we don't touch those stiff-with-dirt hand towels – you haven't a clue who's been using them. Otherwise, just shake your hands dry.

The final hurdle is opening the outer door – all your hand hygiene can be ruined if the person before you hasn't washed their hands before touching it. Use the tip of a finger (or a tissue) to barely touch the handle and out you go. What a relief to be back in the open air!

**APPLIANCE OF SCIENCE**

* Around 20 per cent of women and 40 per cent of men don't wash their hands after using a public loo.
* The toilet seat and the paper towel dispenser in a public loo are likely to have more bacteria on them than the flush handle, the taps or the inside door handle.
* Harmful bacteria can live for up to 17 days on wooden toilet seats.

# Feet

Your feet are your body's major bacterial breeding ground. Shoes don't let the air circulate to cool things off, so moisture builds up until your feet are wringing and minging. Ooh, the cheesy smell when those socks come off. The moist little nooks and crannies between the toes are prime sites for flesh-rotting, fungal nasties such as athlete's foot. Any hard skin on the bottom of your feet gets soggy when your feet sweat, giving bacteria the go ahead to feed and breed and generally pong the place out. Just as well help is at hand. Follow our feet-washing rules and you'll soon be a quick-stepping queen of clean.

# How to wash your feet

Don't be a mucky pup underfoot. Wash your feet at least once a day, more often in hot weather or when you've been standing up all day. A quick freshen-up takes two minutes, and goodness, your nearest and dearest will thank you for it.

Fill a basin with warm, clean water. Dilute a little tea tree oil (from health food shops) in the water if you have some. Tea tree oil has antibacterial properties.

Dunk one foot into the basin and wash with soap. Pay particular attention to the areas between the toes and under the toenails, where nasties lurk.

Rub any areas of rough skin with a pumice stone and rinse well.

Dry the foot thoroughly, especially between the toes.

Repeat with the other foot.

Put on a pair of clean socks (preferably either cotton or natural fibre) and congratulate yourself on a job well done.

**APPLIANCE OF SCIENCE**
* There are around 600 sweat glands per square centimetre on the soles of each foot – that's about 250,000 sweat glands per foot squirting sweat all day.
* Athlete's foot is a highly contagious fungal infection that feeds on dead skin and affects 15 per cent of the population.
* Seriously sweaty feet can be treated with injections of botulinum toxin – but it's both painful (due to the 70,000 or so nerve endings per foot) and expensive.

# Face

Treat the skin on your face gently, or you'll get a hide as tough and wrinkled as an elephant's. In the morning wash with water, but at night the face needs a more generous clean to get make-up and accumulated grime off. We don't like to use body soap on the face – it's too drying – so try a gentle cleanser or wet wipes instead.

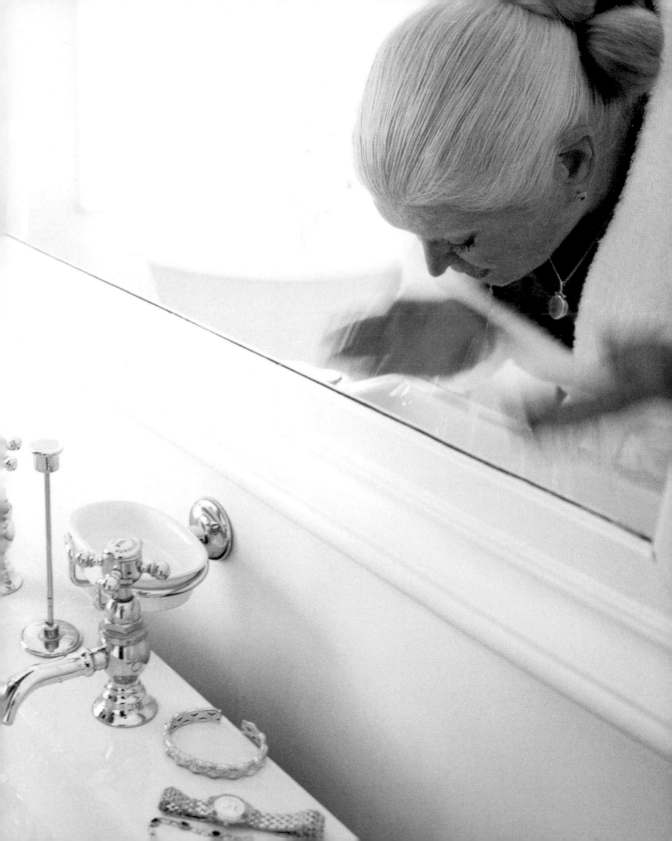

## How to wash your face

Don't go mad – twice a day is enough. We like a two-in-one cleanser that can take off eye make-up too. Saves time and money.

**1** First wash your hands, so that you aren't transferring bacteria to your face.

**2** Use a cleanser appropriate to your skin type. Take a small blob and gently smooth upward over the whole face and eye area in small circular motions. Use your middle and ring fingers rather than your index finger – you won't tug the skin as much.

**3** Leave on for 30 seconds, then rinse well.

**4** Pat skin dry with a clean towel.

Aggie says: 'If you're like me and can't leave spots alone, make sure you don't scar your skin. Steaming your face over a hot bowl of water with a towel over your head for 10 minutes opens the pores in preparation. Then you can extract with minimal damage.'

# What's your skin type?

Before you can get a proper skincare routine going, you need
to determine your skin type.

## Dry skin

Your skin has small pores, is prone to
flaking and feels tight after you wash it.
*What to use:* Don't use soap. Instead,
use a fragrance-free cleanser containing
glycerin that washes away with water.
Avoid toners too – most contain
alcohol which strips oils from the skin.
Moisturise skin in the morning and use
night cream when skin feels dry.

## Oily skin

It often looks shiny and pores tend
to be large. You'll be prone to spots
and breakouts.
*What to use:* It's tempting to use
facial paint-stripper but don't.
Choose a gentle cleanser twice a day.
If you're prone to acne breakouts, try
an antibacterial face wash. You might
like to freshen up during the day
with a mild, alcohol-free toner – try
rosewater or witch hazel. You probably
won't need to moisturise, except
on the neck.

## Normal skin

It's neither dry nor oily. Lucky thing!
*What to use:* Gel cleansers rinse off
easily and don't leave much residue
on the skin. Use a light moisturiser in
summer and a heavier duty one in cold
weather, when skin feels drier.

## Combination skin

This is the most common skin type. You'll
have oily skin around the forehead, nose
and chin – the T section – but normal
to dry skin on the rest of the face.
*What to use:* If your skin looks oily, wash
both morning and night with a gentle,
water-soluble cleanser suitable for
combination skins. During the day, use
rosewater or an alcohol-free toner to
swipe the central greasy patches.
Moisturise daily on cheeks and neck.

# Cheap treats

You don't need to buy expensive facemasks or facials. You've got all the ingredients you need in your kitchen cupboards to give skin a zing.

### Exfoliating skin wash
Grind two tablespoons of dry oats in a coffee grinder – rolled or instant, it makes no difference. Mix in a blender with two tablespoons of honey to make a facial wash. Massage into skin, then rinse off.

### Cucumber facial for normal to oily skin
Mash up half a cucumber and add enough natural live yoghurt to make a paste. Apply thickly to skin, put a couple of cucumber slices over your eyes and relax for 20 minutes. Rinse off with warm water.

### Cream for flaky, irritated skin
Aqueous cream is a bit of a find. It's a bargain (from pharmacies) and moisturises and re-hydrates even the sorest skin.

### Egg facial for combination skin
Break an egg, separate the egg white and yolk, and beat both gently. Place the egg white on the greasy T section of the face, and the egg yolk on drier areas. The white tightens, and the yolk moisturises.

### Peach facial for dry skin
Purée a peach and mix with almond or olive oil to make a smooth paste. Apply to skin and relax for 20 minutes. Rinse off with warm water followed by a cold rinse.

### Sensitive skin treat
Cut a banana into slices, put it into the blender with one tablespoon of honey and mix until smooth. Apply to face and leave on for 20 minutes, then rinse. The honey softens skin, and the banana firms it up, so it's two in one.

### Myrrh massage for mature skins
Mix two drops of myrrh oil into a teaspoonful of almond or wheatgerm oil (all from health food shops). Warm the mixture in the palm of the hand, then gently massage into skin. This is very rich and soothing.

**STAR TIP**
You can't beat witch hazel for toning skin. Pat it on with a cotton wool ball. It has antiseptic properties so even if skin is spotty it's safe to use.

# Soap: what's best?

We like a nice bar of plain toilet soap to wash the hands and body, although moisturising soap is good for dry skin. Not too smelly, mind, or it can be overpowering.

People are always asking us if antibacterial and anti-microbial soaps are worth buying. Well, they're jolly pricey and a bit drying on the hands, we've found. They may be powerful enough to kill bacteria and viruses, but they also strip away protective oils from the skin, leaving it rough and prone to infection. Who wants that? So unless you have older folk or a newborn around the house, whose systems are more vulnerable to germs, we'd say you don't need them. Plain soap is tried and tested and gets most of the bugs off nicely.

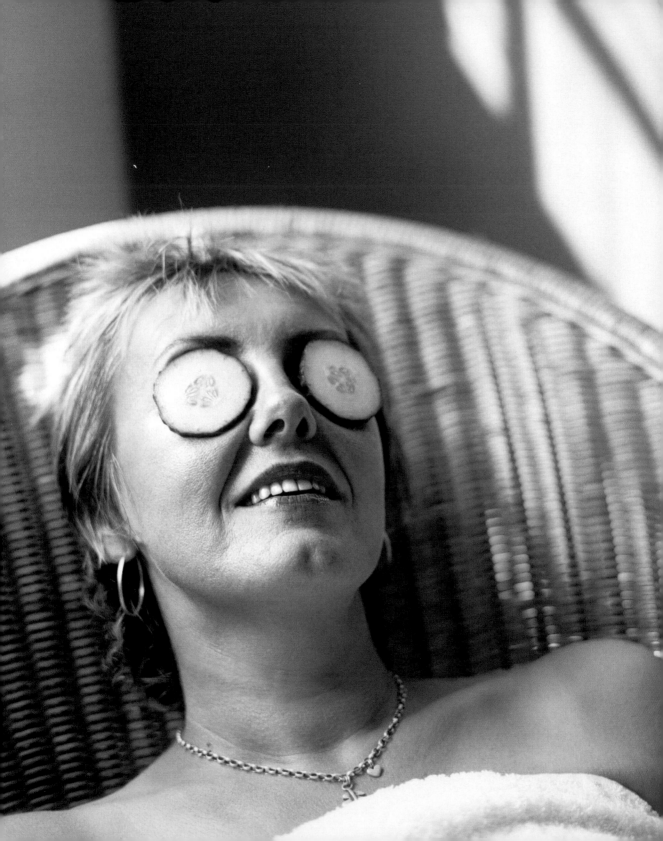

# Aggie's daily routine

I shower daily and occasionally twice daily if I'm going out in the evening or I've had a particularly hard or sweaty time. I can't get going until I've had a shower – I'm completely distracted. I like very hot showers too – my husband always says, 'How can you stand it?' when he comes in afterwards and the bathroom is steamed up like the inside of a kettle.

I don't need a power shower, just lots of hot water and I'm in and out in three minutes. Then a two-minute tooth brush, put moisturiser and make-up on, and I'm ready.

At night, I don't do any of that nonsense with separate eye-make-up remover. I use cucumber-scented face wipes. They have a lovely fresh smell. I find that the first one gets the bulk off, and the second gets everything else off, even clogs of mascara.

My teeth are white but they're in a terrible state underneath. I remember as kids, my sisters and I used to sit on the back step with sticks of rhubarb and a bowl of white sugar and work our way through it. No wonder my teeth are full of fillings. At night it's another two-minute tooth brush. I give it a good go. When I remember I take a dental stick to the plaque.

I like a good slathering of night cream before bed. I put loads and loads on, so it's sitting in big fat layers on my face. My hope is that it's smoothing out all the wrinkles and lines below. Psychologically, if nothing else, it's good for you.

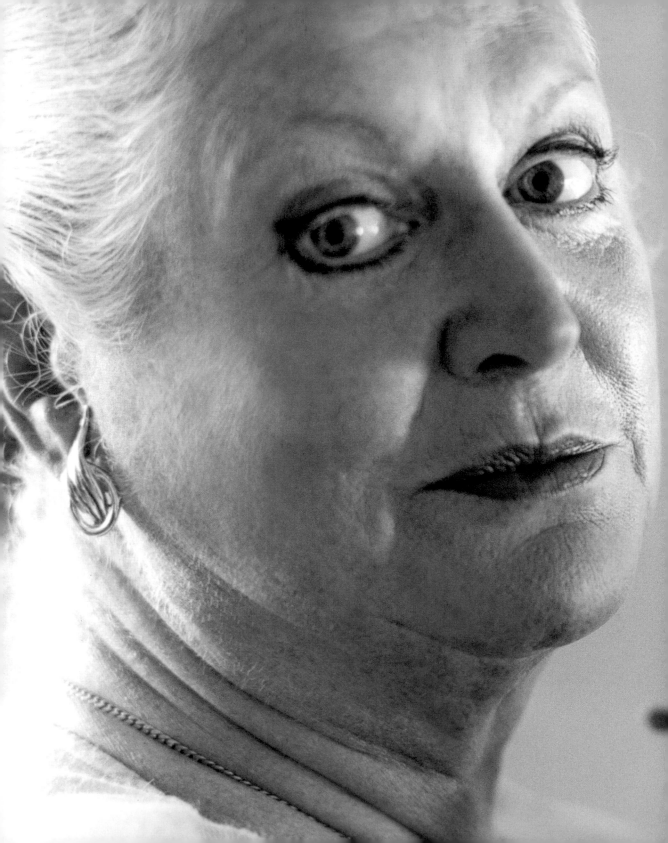

# Kim's daily routine

Ooh, I love to lie in and rot – I have done since I was a young girl. First thing, when I get up, I brush my teeth. After a night's sleep you've got stale breath, stomach acid and whatnot in the mouth. I give my teeth another quick brush after munching breakfast, buffing up with a whitener as well. Before I go out, I take a bubble bath, showering off the soap well. Every two days I wash my hair. It's very dry, so I use lots of conditioner.

I use a moisturiser on my face which helps the make-up flow on better. First I put on foundation, being careful to not let it touch my hairline. Then I do my hair. It takes me 10 minutes, or 15 on a rough day, and I use hair spray to keep it tidy and in place. Then I finish my face off. I always slap on the full works – I think it looks glamorous.

At night, I might have another bath with a few bubbles or just a wash. I always brush the hairspray out of my hair. I take off my make-up with face wipes – they're wonderful. Half an hour before bed I put on moisturiser again, to give it time to sink in. If you've got dry skin like mine, you can feel your skin drinking it in and thanking you for it. Then I brush my teeth and it's off to bed.

# Daily routines

Do the following cleaning routine every day, and you'll be a guaranteed pong-free zone. Your skin and hair will reward you by looking clean, glowing and healthy – and your friends will adore the new sweet-smelling you.

Take a five-minute shower with a bar of soap every morning, come rain or shine.

Dry yourself, making sure every nook and cranny is moisture-free.

If you're clean-shaven, shave daily. No nasty stubble, thank you. Ladies – don't forget to remove your stubble too!

Put on an underarm antiperspirant after showering.

Put on clean undies every day.

Always wash your hands with soap after you go to the loo and before preparing or eating food.

Comb or brush your hair every morning, and as necessary throughout the day.

Take off make-up and wash your face before bed, otherwise bacteria and sebum accumulate causing blackheads and spots.

Brush your teeth for two minutes twice a day, once in the morning and once before bed. Derren, our microbiologist, recommends cleaning for three minutes. And if you can brush them throughout the day, so much the better.

Floss teeth. We know it's easy to forget but just smell all that nasty plaque that comes out!

# Weekly routines

Of course, there are many jobs you don't need to do every day. We can't be spending every minute grooming ourselves. But get yourself a nice system going for the bigger jobs or you'll be in a heck of a mess. Do one or two of these things along with your daily routine and you'll soon be transformed from vagrant to fragrant.

Wash your hair at least once a week. If, like Aggie, yours is short, you may like to wash it every day, but most people only need do it a couple of times a week. Nominate the days for it, so you don't forget.

Have an oily bath. It's good for skin and a weekly soak is relaxing too.

Stimulate circulation with a dry skin brush. Before getting into the bath, use a short-haired bristle brush and rub in circular movements over your whole body – including the soles of your feet. It only takes five minutes and it leaves skin lovely and soft.

Tidy up your eyebrows and other areas where you notice stray hairs. Men should trim their beards at least once a week.

Check your toenails and fingernails and cut if needed.

Moisturise all over with body lotion. We love one that matches our perfumes, but fragrance-free ones are best if you have sensitive skin.

Hand cream is a necessity in all weathers. Massage hand cream in a couple of times a week, or whenever hands feel rough and dry.

Wash your hairbrushes and combs (see page 81).

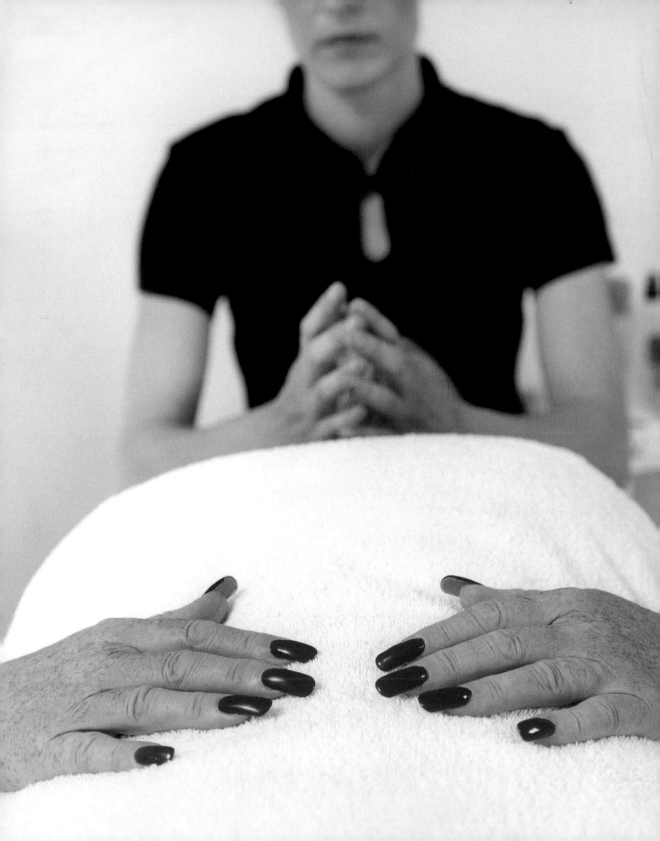

# Regular routines

These little extra things only take a few minutes every so often, but will give you a high-maintenance gloss.

Treat yourself to a home manicure and pedicure (see pages 119 and 122) and check for athlete's foot and other nasties while you're there.

Exfoliate skin all over the body with a home-made scrub (see page 45).

Steam clean your face or use a face mask or home facial to give skin a monthly lift.

Wax or sugar your legs if you prefer not to shave them.

Give feet a treat with a deep moisturising cream applied before you go to bed. Pop a pair of cotton socks over them and when you wake up your feet will be soft as a baby's bottom.

Clean shaving equipment thoroughly and chuck out any scuzzy old blades that are lurking at the back of your bathroom cabinet.

Get your hair cut and styled.

If you colour your hair, you'll need top ups a few times a year. Shampoo-in home treatments will need re-doing too.

We love a body massage – what a treat! If you can't afford a professional, do bits yourself or ask a gentle friend to have a go.

Clean out your make-up bag. Chuck out any mascara you've been using for more than six months – it can harbour nasties.

Clean make-up brushes with a little washing-up liquid or shampoo. Rinse and leave to dry thoroughly in the open air.

Get yourself a new toothbrush. It only takes two to three months before it's skanky.

Once a year, visit the dentist for a check-up. Some folks we know like to get their teeth cleaned by a hygienist every few months too.

BITS
AND
PIECES

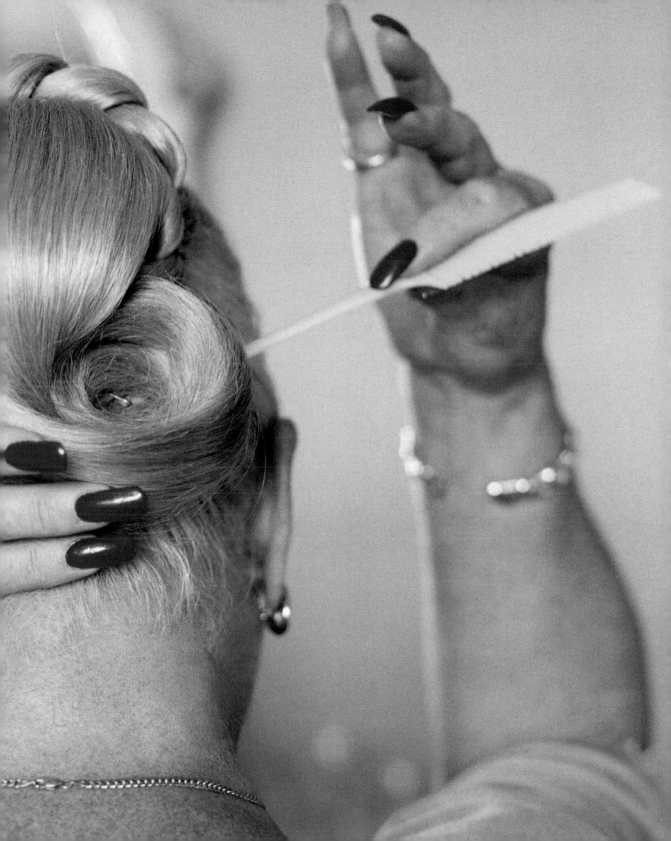

We had a treat on our travels, getting down and dirty and sorting out the personal hygiene of the nation's smelliest beggars. You wouldn't believe how fast we turned them from vagrant into fragrant. With a trim here and a spruce there, even the shaggiest ones came out looking dandy in no time at all.

Taking care of yourself doesn't need much time or money. Nowadays you see posh hair parlours and fancy nail bars on every street corner. But why waste your hard-earned money? You can do most of it yourself, for peanuts.

Grooming is all about maintenance. You have to pay attention to all your bits and pieces. No use having sparkling clean teeth with a lank, filthy mop of hair, now is it? You may look a treat, but if your breath can knock a person down at three paces you're not doing yourself any favours.

# What's that smell?

There are five bits of your body that are most prone to pong:
the underarms, groin, feet, mouth and tummy button. But what
causes the smell?

### Body odour

There are millions of sweat glands all
over the body pumping out body brine
to keep us at the right temperature.
Most of this sweat is salty, and
evaporates without causing too much
of a whiff. But in the primeval hairy bits
under the arms and around the genitals,
the sweat is more potent and bacteria
feast on it causing the unholy pong that
we call body odour. The more someone
sweats, the more likely they are to have
BO, so constant vigilance is needed.

### Bad breath

Those nasty little bacteria are at it
again, causing a right reek. There can be
over 20 varieties at work in your mouth,
stinking the place out. They hide in tiny,
dark cavities on the tongue and
between the teeth and gums. When
they break down proteins in the mouth,
they cause foul smelling gases. And
what a honk they create! They smell of
decaying flesh and rotten eggs. So keep
that pongy little lot under control, dear,
for the sake of the rest of us.

### Tummy button fluff

This is a mixture of dead skin flakes,
fabric from clothes and bacteria. The
tummy button is a nice warm spot that
rarely sees daylight, so bacteria breed
away in comfort, producing black horns
of dense nose-like pickings. The whiff is
awful! 'Innies' harbour more gungy stuff
than 'outies'. You can pick it out with
tweezers – ooh, it's satisfying when it
comes out in one big lump. But be
careful not to pinch your flesh, or skin
can get infected.

### Stinky feet

More of the same bacteria, more of the
same stink. Though this time with a bit
of honking old Camembert on top.
That's thanks to nasty fungi like
athlete's foot, which feeds on rotting
and dead flesh in the damp, dark spaces
between the toes. They cause a right
rotten pong!

# Radiant hair care

Of course, you may want go a mile further than merely washing.
Try some of these treatments.

### To deep condition hair

Good for coloured and blow-dried hair.
Comb mayonnaise through hair, put
on a shower cap and leave for an hour.
Wash out well. Or use two whisked egg
yolks mixed with a tablespoon of olive
oil instead.

### For a good shine on dry hair

Rinse hair in a mix of beer and vinegar.
The beer adds lustre to the hair and
the vinegar adds shine and takes off
shampoo residue. Using a final vinegar
rinse will put the shine back on to
any hair.

### To enhance the colour of hair

Blondes can rinse in an infusion of
chamomile tea and leave in for 10
minutes. Redheads, try rosehip tea.
Brunettes, strong black tea. You can
even sip a cup while you're waiting.

### For natural streaks in blonde hair

Mix a cup of half lemon juice, half water,
apply to hair and go out into the sun. It
will go a lovely golden shade and you've
avoided harsh dyes and bleaches.

### To camouflage grey hair

Try a sage rinse. Make a strong sage
tea using finely chopped fresh sage.
Rinse through hair and leave on for
15 minutes. Rinse out well.

### To manage curly hair

You can apply a smidgeon of KY jelly
to damp hair.

### To moisturise dry, overprocessed hair

Mix 2 tablespoons of mashed avocado
with a quarter cup of mayonnaise. Comb
through hair then cover with a plastic
bag underneath a hot towel. Leave on
for 30 minutes then shampoo as usual.

### To brighten dull hair

If hair looks dull, it could be due to a build up of shampoo residue. Wash as normal, then rinse with one part lemon juice to three parts water.

### To get rid of split ends

Get your hair cut every three months. It doesn't have to be in a salon, a friend can do it for you.

### Dreadlocks

Dirty dreads are a haven for filth and bacteria. Often they're left unwashed for months or even years at a time – we found five million bacteria per gram of hair in one filthy fellow's dreadlocks, 5,000 times more than you'd expect. Imagine the honky smell! But what's worse is that every time you touch dirty dreads, the bacteria transfers to hands – and then everything and everyone you come into contact with is at risk of infection and illness. Keep dreads clean or they can take a serious toll on health! Specialist stylists advise washing dreads every two to three months with a deep conditioning shampoo and conditioner. Wax dreadlocks every two to three weeks with beeswax. Blow dry, and the wax will melt into the hair, keeping it clean and conditioned.

### Low maintenance option

If you really can't be bothered to look after your hair, get a number two buzz cut. It looks good on men or women. You can do it yourself using home-clippers in front of the mirror. It won't need any maintenance apart from washing, and the cut should last up to three months before it grows unruly.

# Dandruff

There's nothing worse than a greasy snowstorm of scaly scalp flakes on someone's shoulders. In bad cases it colonises people's eyebrows and beards, the poor souls. You see them scratching away all over their head because it's as itchy as anything.

In the olden days, they used to rub boric acid into the scalp to treat dandruff. Now you can buy special shampoos. Our advice is to give them a try to see what suits you.

○ Dandruff is the shedding of clumps of dead skin cells from the scalp. Sometimes these become thick, greasy and yellow, a condition called seborrhoeic dermatitis.

○ People with greasy skin are more likely to suffer from it.

○ It's thought to be linked to the overgrowth of a fungus, *Pityrosporum ovale*, on the scalp. It's often worse in winter than summer, probably because humidity levels are lower in winter.

○ Some lifestyle factors trigger dandruff. A salty, sugary, or spicy diet, too much alcohol, changes in hormone levels, and stress all have an effect.

○ For mild dandruff, look out for shampoos containing zinc or selenium, which help control it. With more obstinate dandruff, consult your pharmacist.

○ Try massaging oil (such as vegetable oil) or conditioner into the roots of your hair to help relieve the dryness of the scalp.

**APPLIANCE OF SCIENCE**
* Hair on the head grows about half an inch every month.
* Hair grows faster in summer, and slower in cold weather.
* You shed about 50 to 100 hairs a day.
* Grey hair is usually finer than other hair on your head.

# Hairbrush care

We found *staphylococci* bugs all over the hairs in the hairbrush of one of our soap-dodgers. This bacteria can cause pus-forming infections in and around in the hair follicles on the scalp and neck. Keep your brushes clean!

○ To remove hair from a brush, use the tail of a comb to loosen it, then sweep over the brush with the comb to pull it off. Place loose hair in the bin.

○ Once a week, wash brushes and combs. Soak in a bowl of cold water with a sterilising tablet to disinfect. Rinse, shake, then leave to dry.

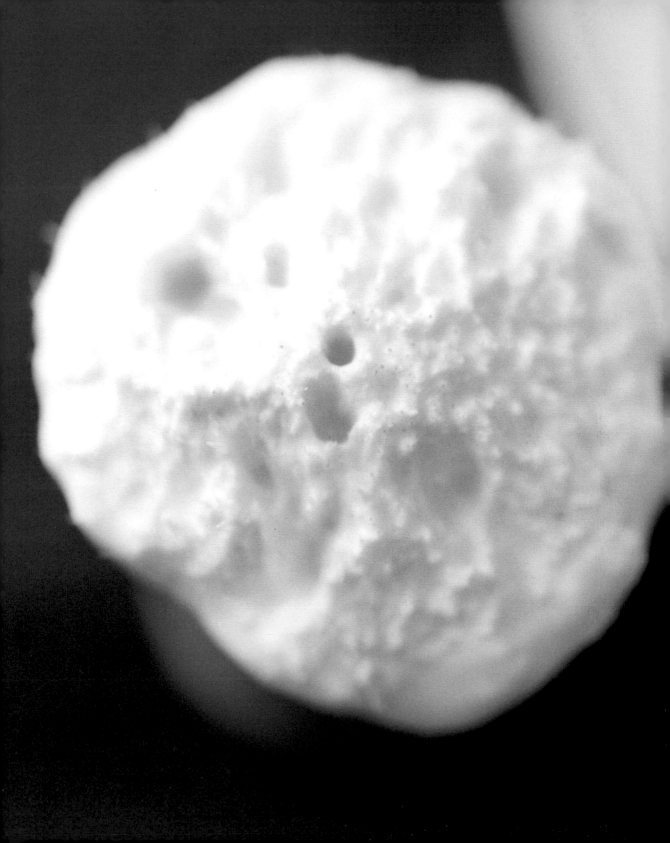

# Shaving

We like a man who wet shaves. We think it's very masculine
and gives the skin a lovely, smooth finish. Still, some men can't
be doing with a wet shave. They come out in rashes and razor
burn or get ingrowing hairs and bumps. An electric shaver can
work wonders for them. It's easier on the skin, though you don't
get such a close cut. But then you can't have everything in one
package, can you?

## Rosewater and vodka aftershave

This is Kim's special concoction. Take 6oml rosewater, 125ml witch
hazel, four teaspoons of vodka, 12 drops of benzoin essential oil,
and four to five drops each of rosemary and geranium essential oils
(all from health food shops). Put into a glass bottle with a stopper,
and shake well. This makes a lovely, fresh, aftershave. The alcohol
will help it keep.

STAR TIP
If you nick yourself
shaving, don't put
tissue on the cut. When
you pull it off the cut
will start bleeding
again. Instead, put a
small blob of shaving
cream on it which
absorbs into the skin.

# Wet shaving routine

It's best to shave after your morning shower or bath, when the pores have opened and the hair has absorbed water and is softer.

**1** Use a shaving soap, gel or foam to lubricate skin and get a good lather up. Leave on for at least a minute before you start shaving to soften hair further.

**2** Rinse your blade in hot water. Then, starting on the cheeks and sides of the face, shave with the direction of hair growth. Although this might not give such a close cut as shaving against the grain, it prevents ingrowing hairs, cuts and razor bumps.

**3** Every two swipes, rinse off your blade with warm water to remove gunk.

**4** Continue shaving the neck, then move on to the upper lip and chin area, where hairs are denser.

**5** When you've finished, rinse with warm water, then splash cold water on the face. Pat dry with a towel. Rinse the blade well before you put the razor away.

# Wet blade care

We found *staphylococcus aureus* on the blade and debris from one of our honker's razors. This bacterium can cause many skin infections including impetigo, which can spread nastily around the face and is highly contagious. If you cut yourself with a dirty blade, you can be infected by your own skin debris. This could cause septicaemia or blood poisoning, which is potentially fatal.

- You need a sharp blade to shave well. A dull blade takes off more skin, leading to irritation, rashes and infection. Change your blade as soon as it is dull, usually every two to five shaves.

- Don't wipe your blade with a towel: it blunts it instantly.

- Always rinse blades in cold water after use.

**APPLIANCE OF SCIENCE**
The average man has around 15,000 whiskers on his face. Facial hair grows about five to six inches a year.

# Electric shaving routine

This doesn't give such a close shave, but heavy-handed clunkers are less likely to lacerate themselves doing it. Good for sensitive skins, and it's not such a palaver as wet shaving so it's worth trying if you're in a hurry.

**1** Only shave on dry skin. Shave in the direction of hair growth. Use a light touch and work with the razor.

**2** Don't dig the heads into your face or you'll cut yourself.

**3** Splash cold water on the face afterwards and apply a slick of moisturiser.

**4** Clean inside the head of the shaver after every use. That's what those little brushes are for.

# Facial fuzz

Call us naïve but we were shocked at some of the hirsute honkers we came across. They had beards because they were too lazy to shave – but they couldn't be bothered to wash or trim their beards, either. Ugh, the sight of those wild and woolly appendages! You could see breakfast, lunch, dinner and other gunky unmentionables hiding in there. Not very Cary Grant, is it?

It doesn't take much to have a neat beard. You can spruce yourself up in two minutes a day. So get your clippers out, lads, and no messing.

**1** Wash your beard in the shower every morning. Boils and furuncles can infect the hair follicle and they love nothing more than dirty, sweaty, hairy skin.

**2** Use conditioner on your beard whenever you wash your hair.

**3** Trim your beard every week. Get a magnifying mirror and hair clippers, and cut to the required length, turning the clippers to work with your hair growth.

**4** Shave any facial and neck areas not covered by your beard.

**APPLIANCE OF SCIENCE**
If beards are not properly maintained, they can become the perfect habitat for a variety of blood sucking human lice. Neglected beards can smell just as bad as armpits – hardly surprising, as they contain the same, acrid-smelling bacteria.

# Bald as a coot?

Shaving your head is not for lazy types. You'll need to redo it every couple of days, depending on hair growth. But if you want to have a go it can look a treat. Just don't say we didn't warn you.

First, cut hair back to a rough stubble with hair clippers.

Shave after a shower when hair has been wet for a few minutes.

Apply shaving soap or gel and leave on for a minute.

Start shaving at the sides and always work with the grain of the hair. Use long strokes.

Move on to the back of the head. This can be tricky. Use a mirror to check you haven't missed any bits.

If you want a very close shave, go over the area again, this time against the grain. You will need to be prepared for this, because it can irritate like billyo.

Rinse off shaving gunk and apply soothing moisturiser. If your scalp is dry, moisturise every day.

**STAR TIP**
If you shave your underarms, it stings when you put your deodorant on. Have a hand towel standing by, and gently beat your stinging underarms with it until the sting disappears.

# Shaving your legs

The same principles apply here as for shaving faces. Electric razors don't give you such a close shave but they are less ruinous for skin. Wet shaving can give you razor burn, ingrowing hairs and other nasties. But then legs are smoother. Up to you, really.

If wet shaving, do it in the bath or shower when legs have been wet for a few minutes. Hair absorbs water, so it will be softer and easier to cut. Use shaving cream or gel rather than regular soap. Only go over skin once, or you risk razor burn. And try not to cut yourself. Blood streaming down your legs is not an attractive look.

Smooth legs need shaving every day – you're lucky if you've got that much time in the morning. Ags can't bear stubble, so she uses an electric tweezer which pulls out the hairs by the roots. Otherwise, there's always waxing. You can do this at home, but it's much nicer to get it all done and dusted in a salon, we think.

Aggie says 'I once had my underarms waxed. It was like giving birth to oversized twins.'

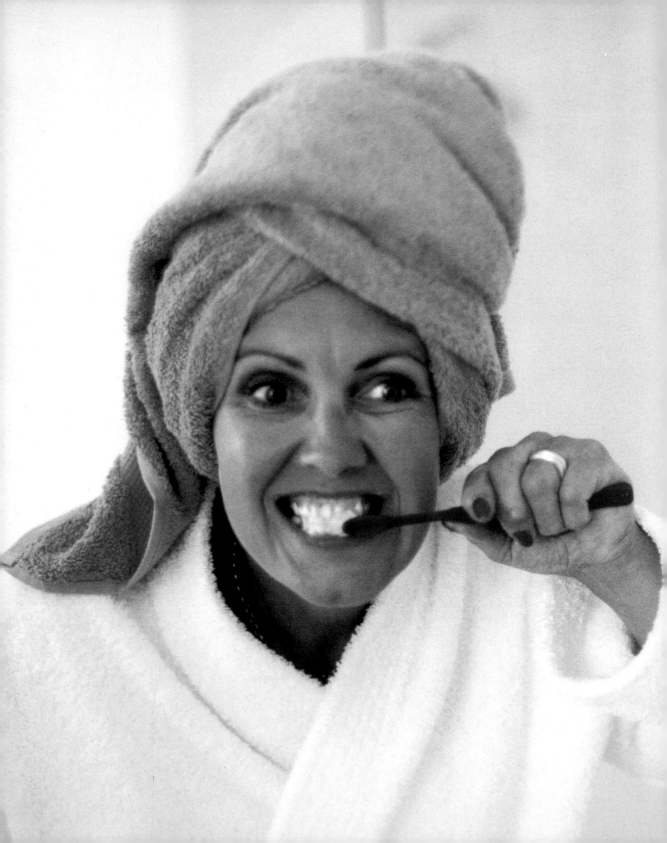

# Open wide!

Horrendous hairy tongues, rotting green-furred teeth
and stonking breath – there are some odorous oral
cavities out there. Every little putrefying scrap of food
left in your mouth is a feast for bacteria, a reservoir for
germs. And ooh, the stench of it! When our soap-dodgers
opened their mouths, we had to run for cover.

But it's not always the teeth that cause the problem.
Most people have up to ten million bacteria in their
mouths. Lots of honky halitosis comes from the tongue,
where bacteria breed and multiply in all the little cracks
and crevices. If teeth are rotten, of course you need to see
a dentist. But otherwise it's down to good oral hygiene.
And we know who's in charge of that, don't we?

bits and pieces

# How to check if you've got bad breath

Do this test: stick your tongue out as far as it will go. Then touch the inside of your wrist to your tongue as far back on your tongue as you can. Wait for ten seconds, then smell. If there's a nasty whiff, there's your answer.

# Why you get bad breath

You don't brush your teeth often enough. You don't clean the spaces between your teeth. Meat and other bits get stuck there and putrefy within hours.

You're a mouth breather, which dries out the mouth. Smoking, fasting, dieting, sleeping, some medications, and anxiety all dry out the mouth, too.

You've got gum disease, plaque, calculous or tooth decay. People with gum disease are three times more likely to have bad breath. See your dentist if your gums bleed when brushing. And start flossing.

If your teeth and gums are healthy, then your tongue is probably the source. Bacteria easily gets trapped on the tongue, and breeds prolifically. Brush your tongue as well as your teeth.

You have a throat infection, catarrh, sinusitis or other related problem. Check with your doctor if you suspect anything other than oral hygiene is to blame.

People with hairy tongues – enlarged papillae on the surface – are more likely to suffer from bad breath.

**APPLIANCE OF SCIENCE**

∗ If you don't brush your teeth, bacteria breed in large numbers, encouraging tooth decay, absesses, gum disease and the erosion of bone in the jaw. Oral infections cause fever, swelling, and can spread to the brain, nearby bones and soft tissue.

∗ The bacteria in the mouth produces foul-smelling compounds such as hydrogen sulphide, methyl mercaptan and putrescine, which smell like rotten eggs, faeces and decaying flesh.

∗ People with gum disease are nearly twice as likely to suffer from coronary heart disease, as the bacteria causes infections of the heart valve. If left untreated the death rate is 100 per cent.

∗ Smokers are more likely to suffer from periodontitis, a tooth disease that affects the gums and bone.

# Toothpaste

You can make your own toothpaste, but frankly what a faff!
Most toothpastes contain fluoride, though if you're anti, you can
buy ones without. Pump-action tubes are less messy than standard
tubes. We can't be doing with those strawberry-flavoured brands –
give us a fresh, minty taste any day.

### Baking soda

This cleans and whitens teeth and
freshens breath. Rub on to teeth with
a brush and a little water, and rinse well.
If you keep baking soda in the bathroom,
store it in a glass jar. A cardboard box
will disintegrate.

### False teeth treatment

If you have dentures and want them
extra clean, brush with a thin layer of
baking soda. Set them to soak in glass of
water with an extra teaspoon of baking
soda added. Leave overnight and they'll
be sparkling in the morning.

### To whiten teeth

Rub ripe strawberries over teeth to give
teeth a sparkling glow. Rinse well.

## Chew on this

Bacteria breeds nicely on a sticky film of plaque which can cover teeth leading to decay and diseases. Derren, our resident microbiologist, says you can check how well you're cleaning your teeth using pink, plaque-detecting disclosing tablets (available from a pharmacist) which stain the plaque red. We tried this on one of the mucky pups on the programme and her teeth came out so red she looked like Dracula's handmaiden.

## Botanical breath fresheners

○ Gargle with the juice of half a lemon diluted with water. Many commercial breath fresheners only mask the smell for 10 or so minutes. They contain alcohol which dries out the mouth and can make the problem worse.

○ Rinse your mouth after eating dairy products, fish and meat. Protein-rich foods encourage bacteria.

○ Chew parsley after meals, especially after eating garlic or strong-smelling foods. It's nature's own deodoriser.

○ Chew on a clove. It has anti-bacterial properties. Clove oil can soothe toothache, too.

○ Chew sugar-free gum for a few minutes every so often: it helps you produce more saliva which washes bacteria away.

# Don't waste water
Leaving the tap running while brushing teeth or shaving can waste around three gallons of water a minute. Better to turn the tap off.

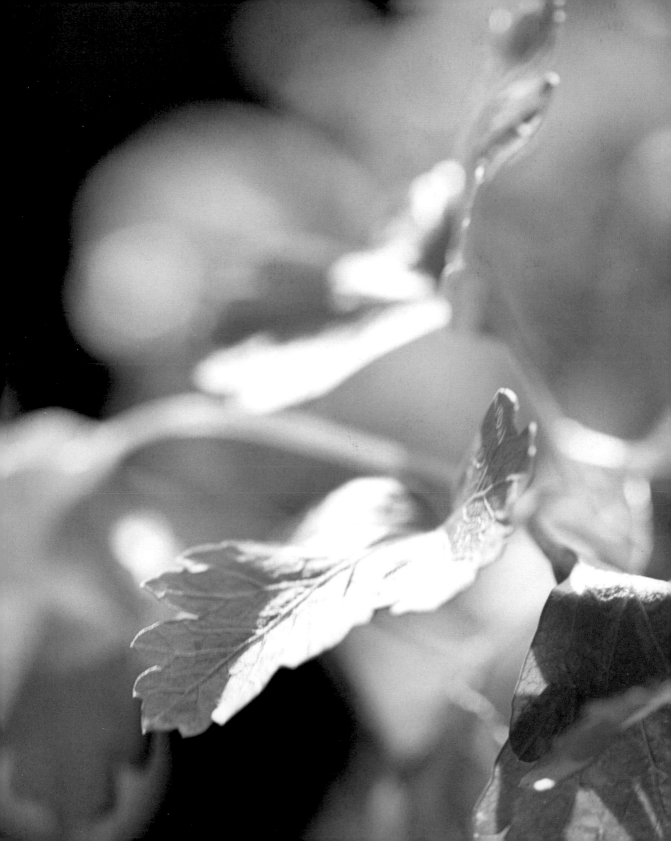

# Eyes

They say they're the window to the soul, but goodness they take a beating. If you're the least bit tired they look all saggy, baggy and bloodshot.

## Bright eyes botanically

Blink more often to avoid dry, itchy eyes.

For bright, healthy eyes: dampen two cotton wool balls with Eyebright solution (available from health food shops) and wipe eyes every few hours.

To reduce swelling and puffiness: place an infused tea bag over each eye and relax for ten minutes.

Eat your cabbage, broccoli, carrots and peas. You'll be healthy with all those vitamins and your eyes will thank you.

## Contact lens care

You shouldn't choose contact lenses unless you are prepared to look after them properly. We found the deadly bacteria *Serratia* in one of our soap-dodger's contact lens cases. This can cause *microbial keratitis*, an infection of the cornea which can lead to loss of sight and even blindness.

1 Don't lick contact lenses to lubricate them. Saliva contains millions of bugs that can cause conjunctivitis and other infections. Use re-wetting drops instead.

2 Even bottled water is a no-no for washing lenses. It can contain water-based bacteria such as *pseudomonas* and *Serratia*, and parasites such as Acanthamoeba. These breed on the lens and on the eye, damaging the cornea.

3 Avoid mascara with lash-extending fibres which irritate around the contact lens. Don't use glitter eye shadow either.

4 Don't use home-made saline solutions to clean lenses as you risk infection.

5 Wash hands before handling lenses. Put a clean towel underneath when you handle lenses. Then if you drop them, they don't get lost, filthy or scratched.

**STAR TIP**
For puffy eyes in the morning, pat haemorrhoid cream under the eye. It shrinks the skin and the puffiness disappears fast.

# Ears

Ears do best when they are left well alone. Don't be poking your finger in there, or you'll cause infection. Give a good scrub behind your ears every time you wash your hair and that should do it. Otherwise, our ear care is really a list of don'ts, rather than dos. When it comes to ears, less is more.

## Ear care

○ Don't even think about pushing fingers, cotton wool buds, paper clips, hairgrips or anything else into ears. They can compact wax and break the skin, giving bacteria and fungi a foothold. However, do wipe gently around the outer part of the ear with a damp flannel.

○ If you have hairs growing out of your ears, please give them a good prune every so often and do us all a favour.

○ Don't use a towel to dry your ears. Instead, use a hair dryer on a gentle setting. Or just leave well alone.

○ Showering, bathing and swimming can cause swimmer's ear, a painful infection caused by dirty water trapped in the ear. These eardrops can help: put two to three drops of a 1:1 solution of surgical spirit and clear distilled vinegar into the ear. It dries out the ear, stopping bacterial growth.

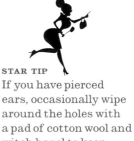

**STAR TIP**
If you have pierced ears, occasionally wipe around the holes with a pad of cotton wool and witch hazel to keep them free from bacteria.

# Underarms

If there's one place you can guarantee that soap-dodgers will pong, it's their underarms. They think that if they don't flap their arms around, the rest of us won't notice the niff. How wrong can they be? Get washing now, you mucky pups, and afterwards have a go at some of these sweet-smelling solutions.

After you apply antiperspirant, give your underarms a whack with a dry towel to take the residue off. Don't wipe, just a couple of strong pats. It keeps the area nice and dry when you put your clothes on.

**STAR TIP**
Wear cotton clothes rather than man-made fibres and keep your jacket on in sweaty situations.

# Antiperspirants vs deodorants

Antiperspirants are designed to stop you sweating by blocking the sweat glands under the arm. Their active ingredients are aluminium or zirconium. Deodorants are designed to mask the smell – but they don't stop you sweating, so you still get damp patches under your arms.

# How to have heavenly pits

Trim or shave underarm hair. Hair traps sweat, giving the bacteria more to munch on.

Underarm antiperspirants and deodorants contain different active ingredients. Try a few until you find one that works for you. You can find deodorants that don't contain aluminium or parabens – chemicals that some believe are linked to breast cancer – in health food shops.

For a herby deodorant, put two drops each of rosemary, cypress and lemon essential oils into a small bottle. Add eight drops each of cedarwood and patchouli essential oils. Add 125ml distilled (must be distilled!) witch hazel and mix together for a wonderful deodorant. Apply with cotton wool.

If you like a natural deodorant, use baking soda. It can sting, so mix half and half with cornflour (or talc, though that often has a fragrance) and apply when underarms are washed but still slightly moist, not dry. It works a treat.

Ammonium alum crystal is a naturally occurring mineral salt with antibacterial properties. Use on wet underarms. It scratches a bit when you put it on, but deters BO (though not sweating). From health food shops.

If you sweat profusely, try an anti-perspirant containing 20 per cent aluminium chloride (from pharmacies). You use it at night, applying on perfectly dry skin before you go to bed. Wash it off in the morning. It stops sweating by swelling the sweat glands, but can be drying and irritating for skin long-term.

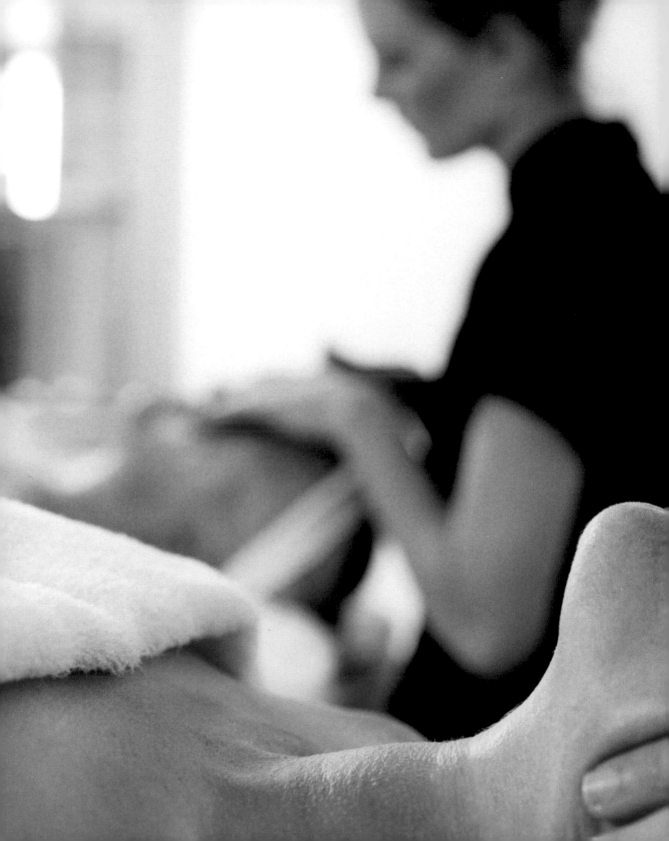

# Blackheads, blemishes and acne

We've certainly seen some pimples, boils and blackheads during our mission to clean up Britain. There's some acne around, we can tell you. We've seen skin erupting in pustules and hard, pus-filled cysts causing awful pain. It breaks your heart to think of the poor dears suffering from these terrible skin afflictions. And it's not just teenagers. It's grown men and women, who surely hoped the spots would have gone by the time the wrinkles had arrived.

Acne has a terrible effect on people's lives. Well, who'd want to be the life and soul of the party with a face full of zits? But there's no need to stay at home and suffer. If your spots are bad enough, see a doctor. Otherwise there are a few things to try.

## What is acne?

Don't believe those old wives' tales that say you get acne from eating chocolate or chips. It's mainly due to hormones and heredity. It's caused by the overproduction of sebum in the sebaceous glands of the skin. When hair follicles get plugged up with this excess oil, bacteria called *Propionibacterium acnes* thrive.

Soon, blackheads and whiteheads form, and inflammation in the blocked follicles can erupt into painful pustules. In the worst cases, you can see pus-filled lumps below the skin. If these rupture, they spread the infection and cause scarring. Acne occurs most often on the face, back and chest, where there are more sebaceous glands per square inch. About 20 per cent of acne cases occur in adults, and women are more likely to suffer than men.

# Gently does it...

# Acne control

Gently is the key word, if you want to get acne under control.

Don't be tempted to scrub acne-prone skin. Instead, wash the face twice a day – no more, please – with a pH balanced cleanser.

Try to resist picking and prodding – it can cause terrible scarring. If there's a pustule you just must squeeze, first warm the area using a clean cloth dipped in hot water. Then pierce it with a needle sterilised under a flame and gently ease out the pus with a tissue.

If skin looks greasy during the day, tone with witch hazel, rosewater (both from pharmacies) or an alcohol-free astringent.

If you use spot concealer, make sure it's medicated. Thick, greasy make-up clogs pores even more.

Apply a gel containing benzoyl peroxide (from pharmacies) to the affected areas twice a day. This kills the bacteria, but it can dry skin out. If it doesn't work in four to six weeks, see your doctor.

**APPLIANCE OF SCIENCE**
Each square inch of skin contains about 20 hairs and 30 sebaceous glands. If just one of these follicles gets infected and ruptures subcutaneously, bacteria spread and acne can take hold.

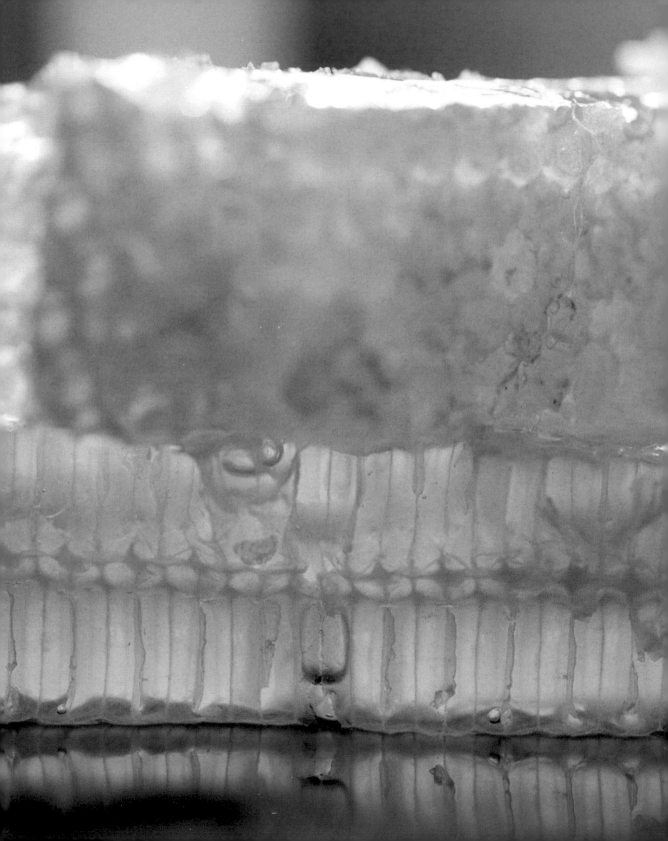

# Anti-acne action

### Gentle exfoliator for blackheads

Mix some runny honey with a little oatmeal and an egg white to form a paste. Rub gently over the skin in circular movements, then leave for 10 minutes. Rinse well. The egg white dries the oil and the oatmeal gently exfoliates skin.

### Tea tree acne treatment

Dab tea tree oil (from health food shops) on affected skin and allow to dry. Tea tree oil has antiseptic and antibacterial properties.

### Aloe vera soother

Acne-prone skin can be very sensitive. As a soother, splash cold water on to the face for 20 seconds, then apply a light coating of cold-processed aloe vera gel (available from health food shops).

### Vitamin E healer

Prick a vitamin E capsule with a pin. Squeeze out and rub into damaged skin to aid healing. If you don't empty the capsule, stand it up and the hole will heal itself so you can use the rest later! Some people are sensitive to vitamin E so before putting it on your face, smear a small amount on the inside of your upper arm and leave for an hour or so to make sure there is no reaction.

# Other bits and bobs

## Mind your make-up

We don't want you getting all obsessive. Everything in moderation. But we've been talking to our lovely microbiologist, Derren, who had some scary things to say about what nasties can be lurking in your make-up.

○ Old make-up provides a perfect breeding ground for bacteria, which can easily be spread around if you share make-up brushes or mascaras. In the eyeliner wand of one of our honkers we found the bacteria that leads to conjunctivitis – a nasty eye infection that causes redness, pus and swelling. This kind of bug can also scar the cornea and lead to loss of vision.

○ Keep mascara in the fridge – it prevents bacteria growing. Only use mascara for six to eight months then chuck it out. It can be riddled with bugs that cause nasty eye infections like conjunctivitis or corneal ulcers.

○ Don't put water or saliva on to your mascara wand or liquid eyeliner. It gives water-based bugs a chance to colonise. If you need to clean the wand, give it a quick wipe with an antibacterial wipe, then put the wand straight back into the tube of mascara.

○ Old foundation can give you bumpy skin. This is caused by an infection in the hair follicle. The worst are those you apply by dipping your finger into the pot. Tube foundations are more hygienic. If you apply foundation with your fingers rather than a sponge, make sure you wash your hands first.

○ Don't share any cosmetics or brushes with anyone, not even your nearest and dearest. You'll just be spreading germs.

○ Make-up can cause blocked pores, so remove before bed.

○ Every couple of months, wash make-up brushes in warm water with a bit of washing up liquid or shampoo. Dry quickly – use a hair dryer if you need to. This gets rid of grease and bacteria.

○ When your powder puff becomes darker than your powder, that's perspiration and grease from the skin. Wash it every couple of weeks, or use tissues instead.

# Pluck the blighters

Aggie says: 'There's something that really annoys me about straggly eyebrows – it's like a sign you're not washing under your armpits. To me, it's basic grooming. I love a good pluck myself. If you're squeamish, an ice cube on the area beforehand can help dull the pain.'

Pluck your eyebrows in natural daylight as you will be able to see stray hairs more clearly.

Take out any stray hairs first, then you can see the natural line of the brow.

Pluck to the required shape, taking hairs out from underneath the brow, never above.

Always pluck hairs in the direction of growth, then they won't stick out when they grow back.

A cotton wool ball soaked in hot water and applied to the brow will help soften and open the pores, making plucking less painful.

# Healthy hints

**Relief for sunburn**
Make a thick paste with two teaspoons of cornflour and some water. This relieves sunburn and itching. If your nose burns badly, lather this on. You won't look your best but it'll relieve your poor nose.

**To counteract poison ivy**
Make a thin paste of powdered milk and water. Spread over the trouble spot to stop itching.

**For cold sores**
You need to be brave for this one. Spray cologne on to a cold sore – it will sting for a minute and a half. Next day, it will feel a lot better.

**For splinters**
If you have a splinter in your finger, put olive oil on it to soften the skin. It can then work itself out with some gentle easing. If not, go in for the kill and be brave!

FOOT AND
HAND NOTES

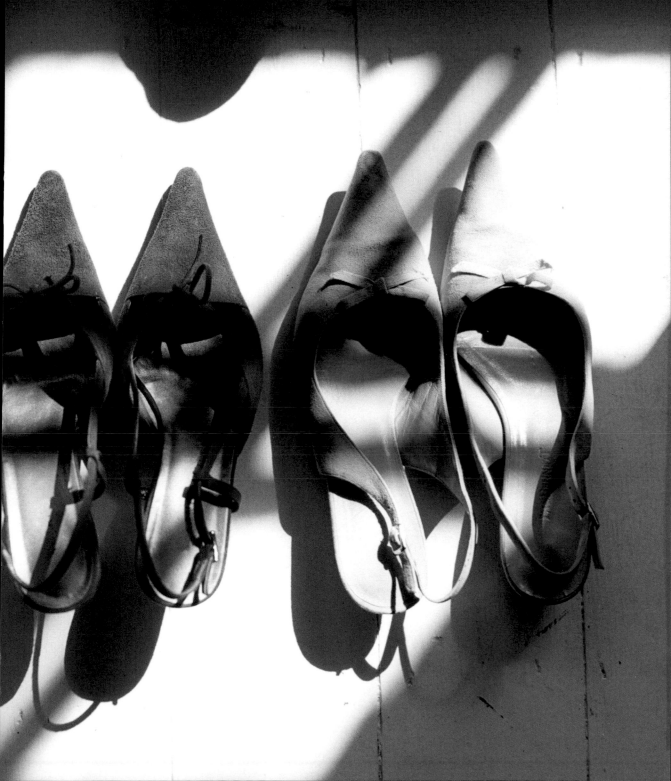

Feet don't half stink. Well, they sweat buckets, and they don't see much daylight either. When was the last time you walked barefoot in the early morning dew? Or even padded around the house without socks or slippers on?

The average person takes 15,000 steps during the 16 hours they're on their feet each day. And it doesn't matter whether you're wearing high heels or trainers, your feet will be lathering up with sweat as nicely as the winner of the Grand National.

Hands sweat too, but it evaporates so quickly that you hardly notice. That's the trouble with feet. When sweat gathers in airless socks and shoes, bacteria and fungi leap into action. Just hours later your toes will be as cheesy as Gorgonzola and an almighty ming will start rising.

Ooh, the honk of the festering feet we've come across along the way. One filthy so-and-so hadn't washed his socks for weeks and had millions of bacteria crawling all over them. There's no excuse for it.

# How stinky
# are your feet?

Yoga aficionados will be able to get
their foot up to their nose for a good sniff.
The rest of us have to be more inventive.

1 Take swabs from between the toes with
a cotton wool bud. If it's honky, you've
probably got athlete's foot.

2 Before bed, smell the sock you've worn
that day. Rate it on a ming factor of one
to ten. Be honest now. Anything over
five and attention is needed.

3 Ask a friend or family member to smell
the inside of your trainers. If they pass
out, you'd better read on.

# Foot diseases

Foot diseases are not fun. It's painful having rotting, disease-ridden flesh deep between your toes. Fungi and bacteria love feet because they're hot, sweaty and rarely see the light of day. These are some of the worst little offenders.

## Athlete's foot

You can pick this fungus up anywhere. Carpets, bedding, swimming pools, changing rooms, showers and towels all harbour it, and it can survive for weeks without a host to feed on.

It loves dark, damp spaces so often starts between toes. Let it get a foothold and tiny blisters develop, causing itching, redness and soft, scaling skin. This can lead to painful cracks and deeper fissures. As the mould rots the skin, there's an almighty pong. It can colonise toenails, which become thick and crumbly. You can also transfer it to your groin or other moist, warm areas of the body through hand contact.

○ Wash feet and put on clean cotton or natural fibre socks every day.

○ Drying feet well reduces the likelihood of athlete's foot developing. Pay special attention to the toe web, and between the fourth and fifth toes.

○ In swimming pools and gyms, wear flip-flops in the shower and changing rooms.

○ If you have athlete's foot, wear cotton socks and, if possible, warm them to help kill the fungi.

○ Use a topical antifungal treatment (from pharmacies).

# Pitted keratolysis

This little bug causes a right reek! It loves nothing more than a hot, sweaty foot trapped inside hot, sweaty trainers. Sporty types who perspire prolifically get it. It causes little white or brown pits in the skin of the sole, especially on the pressure points of the heel, ball of the foot and toe pads. The resulting bacterial stew is very smelly. Pitted keratolysis can transfer on to hands, too.

Wear trainers and boots only when you have to.

Look for trainers that have mesh or cloth sides. These allow feet to breathe a little.

Always shower and wash feet thoroughly after playing sport.

This one loves the damp, so dry feet well after washing, using a hair dryer on the soles.

Never wear shoes without socks, and change socks immediately after sweaty workouts.

Apply spray antiperspirant to feet every day.

In hot weather, wear sandals or open-toed shoes whenever you can. But please, men, give yourself a pedicure first (see page 119).

If all else fails, consult a pharmacist.

# Sweaty feet

One lad we met had the stinkiest feet, poor lamb. You wouldn't believe the sweat that poured out of them all day and every day. He was suffering from excessively overactive feet and his room stank of it. What a king of ming!

Some people just sweat more than others. The name for this is hyperhidrosis, and there's no need to be embarrassed about it. But if you don't want to be a social cripple, you need to tackle the root cause. It's not the sweat that smells, it's the decomposition of bacteria that feed on it. Keeping your shoes and socks pristine clean will help with the pong.

○ Terminally sweaty feet can benefit from a little TLC. Wash feet at least twice a day. We don't like antibacterial soap as a rule. But try it as a last resort if those microbes are still minging.

○ Spray on antiperspirant in the morning, or try the 20 per cent aluminium chloride treatment (see page 99) for a few nights to stop excess sweating.

○ Dusting clean feet with a powder puff of baking soda every morning can help keep the smell down.

○ Try surgical spirit. It cleans off bacteria. Stop using if it irritates or dries skin.

○ After washing and drying feet, wipe with a cotton wool ball soaked in witch hazel or clear distilled vinegar.

○ In severe cases, your doctor might recommend iontophoresis, where a low electric current is passed through the surface of feet, partly blocking the sweat glands. Repeat treatments are needed. Botulinum injections are also a possibility, although these are painful and pricey.

# Dunk your feet, dear!

### Sage and pine foot fresheners

Some people sprinkle garlic powder on their feet but we find sage and pine a little easier on the nasal cavities. Add a few drops of essential oil of sage or pine into a foot bath and soak feet for 10 minutes. You'll soon smell like spring time on a mountainside.

### Fresh foot bath

Add a handful of Epsom salts and a glass of vinegar to a bowl of warm water and bathe feet for 15 minutes. This deodorises and refreshes.

### Lemon foot wash

Lemon deodorises all those nasty nooks and crannies, and lightens and smoothes skin too. Mix the juice of five lemons with a cup of warm water in a shallow foot bath. Stand feet in it for five to 10 minutes. Then rinse off and dry well. One word of warning: don't try this if you have athlete's foot. It'll sting!

### Hot oil soak

Dry feet will benefit from this one. Wash feet, then warm some vegetable oil. When cool enough to touch, pour the oil over feet to half cover them in a shallow foot bath. Rub the oil into the top of each foot with the bottom of the other foot. Give feet a massage. Rinse feet well. Pour the oil into a jar with lid, and you can use it again.

### Rough skin healer

Vegetable shortening – the kind you use for making puff pastry – is wonderful for rough scaly feet. Before bed, rub shortening into the rough patches on feet, then pull on some old socks to protect the sheets. In the morning, your feet will be lovely and soft.

### Natural foot deodoriser

Boil a quart of water, then steep four or five teabags in it. Allow to cool, then pour the tea into a bowl. Soak feet for 30 minutes, and dry off without rinsing. The tannin in tea is a natural astringent.

foot and hand notes

If you've got
real stinkers
at the end
of your legs,
you need to
get washing.

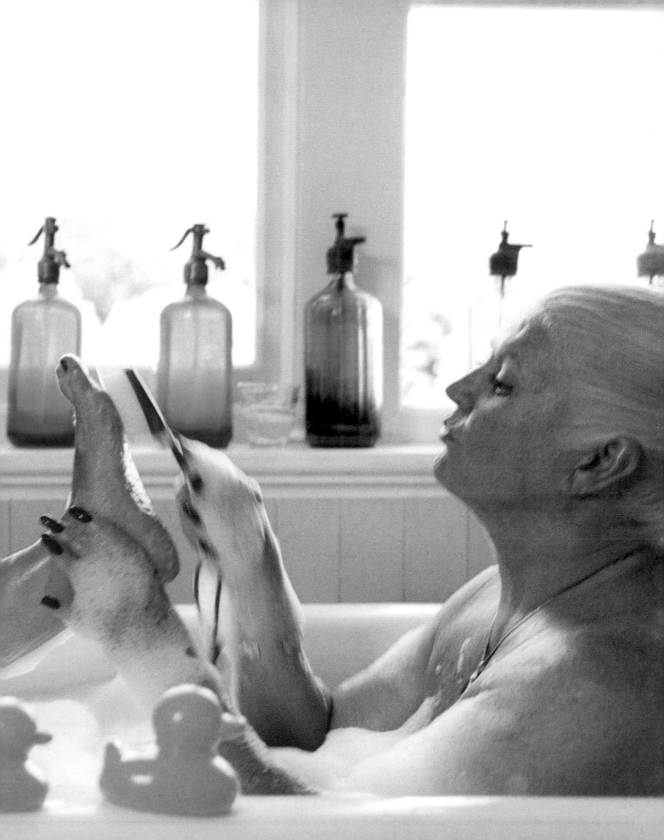

# Stinky shoe care

Choose well-fitting shoes that don't rub or irritate feet. And it's a good idea to de-pong them every so often.

○ Plastic and vinyl shoes collect sweat. Don't save your pennies, go for natural materials like leather or canvas instead. Check the insides of your leather shoes – it won't help the smell if they have a plastic lining.

○ Have two or three pairs of shoes and rotate them daily, so each pair gets the chance to dry out.

○ Wear trainers as little as you can. They are sweat buckets. Wash in the washing machine on a short gentle cycle with a load of old towels (to prevent them banging against the drum) and they come out as good as new.

○ Dab cornflour in your shoes to freshen them up. It absorbs moisture.

○ Put charcoal insoles in your shoes. They eat up odour. Normal insoles cut the sniff factor, too, if you wash them every day.

○ Vacuum the insides of shoes. It sucks out dead skin, dirt and dried sweat.

○ Avoid chucking shoes at the bottom of your wardrobe where they can collect mildew. Let them dry out on racks.

○ Sandals and open-toed shoes let air circulate nicely around the feet. Wear them whenever weather allows.

○ To deaden the niff of stinky shoes, sprinkle bicarbonate of soda liberally into them. Place them in a plastic bag in the freezer for 24 hours. Before wearing, shake the bicarb out.

**STAR TIP**
To freshen up leather shoes, dab tea tree oil on cotton wool and wipe around the inside of the shoes. Leave to dry.

# Stinky sock care

Chuck out your nylon socks. Stock up on those containing 60 to 70 per cent wool or cotton instead. They're a bit pricier but they absorb sweat better. **1**

Change your socks every day. Twice a day if you sweat a lot. **2**

Don't wear socks that are too small. They squeeze your toes and cause sweatiness and rubbing. **3**

Wash cotton socks at 60°C to kill nasties – although always check the care label first. **4**

# Treat your feet

It's once in a blue moon with pedicures, we know. And if truth be told, we can be a bit slack in this area ourselves. But a good home pedicure every month is a treat indeed. Even better if you can bribe someone else to do it for you.

## Aggie's home pedicure

Apply a blob of cuticle cream to the base of each nail and massage gently in.

Soak feet in a bowl of warm water with a tiny squirt of washing-up liquid in it. I like a swish of tea tree oil too. A 10-minute soak should soften them up nicely.

Gently push back cuticles with a cotton wool bud.

Cut toenails straight across to prevent any ingrowing tendency.

Then pick the cheesy bit out of the corner with nail scissors. This is the best bit!

Take your pumice stone and start sloughing off that thick, dead skin on the soles and around the heels. That's a gourmet bacteria breeding ground.

Give yourself a little foot massage. Knead the sole with your knuckles, bend all your toe joints, press your thumbs around your heels and ankle joints. Gently press the soft points on the inside of your big toe. Clears your head nicely, doesn't it?

If you want to paint toenails, dry feet first then put rolled-up tissue between toes to keep them straight (or use a toe-separator, if you have one).

Starting at your little toe to avoid smudging, apply varnish. Recoat if necessary.

When nails are dry, rub a rich moisturising cream into feet.

**STAR TIP**
Go shoe shopping in the afternoon rather than the morning. Feet will be slightly swollen then, and you won't be tempted to buy shoes that are too small. Kim always buys shoes half a size too big to allow for expansion during the day.

# Hands and nails

Hands need a different kind of treatment from feet. They're on show and raggedy unkempt nails and horny skin don't impress anyone. A bit of grooming can work wonders. Give hands a good scrub, manicure, and slather on the cream. They'll spruce up a treat.

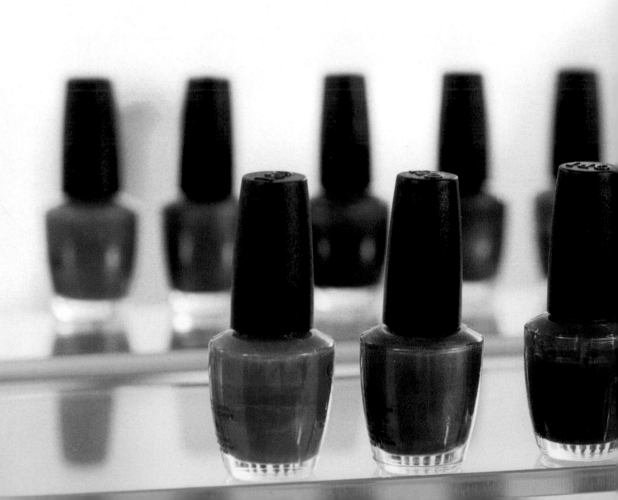

# How to file your fingernails

Nail scissors for feet, but an emery board for fingernails, please. We like the big, wide black ones, that don't bend when you use them.

It's easier to start with your pinkie and work towards your thumb.

Using the rough side of the emery board, shorten the nail to the right length. Don't saw backwards and forwards. File from the outer corners into the centre.

To shape the nail, use the finer side of the emery board. Again, file in one direction only, making sure the edge of the nail is smooth.

Rub a little handcream or baby oil into the nails then gently buff up.

# Have a home manicure

Your hands see you through a lot, don't they? So once a month, lavish some love and attention on those poor digits. We do this one in front of the telly at night so we're not wasting precious cleaning time. It's good after a bath or washing the dishes, too, when your hands will be soft and clean already.

**1** Remove old polish using an acetone-free remover. It's gentler on the nails.

**2** File nails, then blob a bit of cuticle cream (from chemists) over the base of your nails and rub in gently. Soak fingers in a basin of warm water for five minutes. Alternatively, you can soak nails in the beaten yolk of an egg to soften them.

**3** Using a cotton wool bud, push back cuticles and hangnails. Be very gentle. Don't scratch the surface of the nail. Wipe off any excess cream and dry well.

**4** While hands are wet, clean under the nails using an old toothbrush or nailbrush. This is where most of the bacteria lurk.

**5** Apply a clear or base coat to nails if you're using a strong-coloured varnish. It stops the nails getting stained.

**6** Apply the varnish of your choice using three strokes, one in the centre, then one at each side.

**7** Don't flap your hands around to dry varnish – it makes it wrinkle.

**8** Depending on the colour, you may need another coat. Wait until nails are completely dry before applying.

**9** Add a colourless top coat when the varnish is dry, to help prevent nails chipping and to add a lovely shine.

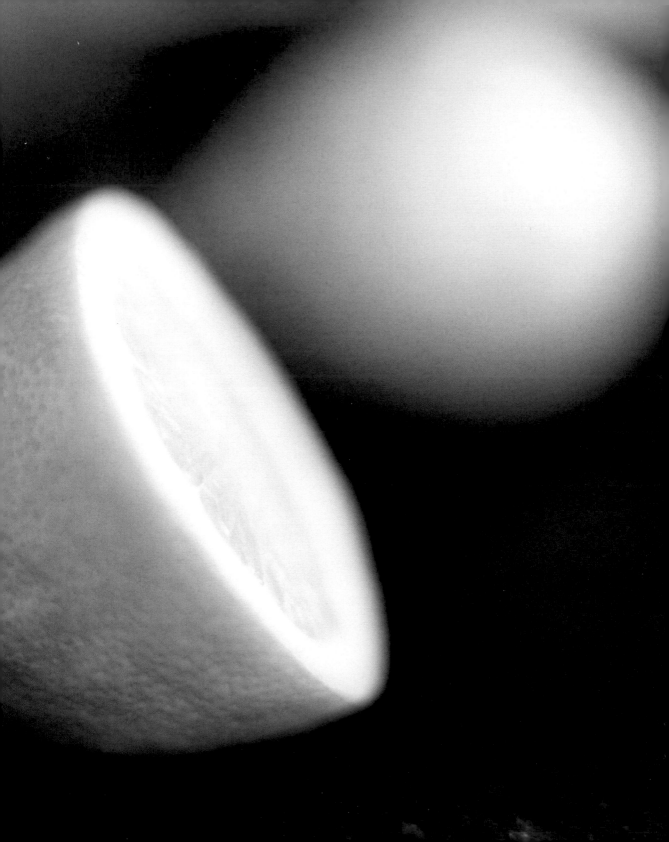

# Natural cures

**Gardening hand scrub**
Mix two heaped teaspoons of sea salt
with enough olive oil to make a paste.
Rub into hands and rinse well. This will
remove grubby gardening stains.

**To remove stains**
Lemon juice works well for stains on the
hands. Dilute the juice of half a lemon in
half a glass of warm water. Soak the hands
for 10 minutes, then rinse and pat dry.

**For sweaty palms**
Dab a little cornflour on to the palms
with a powder puff to keep hands dry.

**For super-smooth mitts**
Before you go to bed, lavish handcream
on your hands. Pull a pair of disposable
white cotton gloves on top. Cheap
and cheerful, and when you wake
up next morning your hands will
be heavenly.

**For dry, scaly hands**
Before bed, rub some vegetable
shortening – the kind you use for
pastry – into hands, pop on some
cotton gloves, and leave overnight.
It's odourless, it costs a fraction of
what you can pay for fancy lotions,
and it works wonderfully.

**For brittle, split nails**
Split nails are dry nails. Soak them
in a finger bowl of warmed olive
or wheatgerm oil for 10 minutes.
Massage the oil gently into nails
and cuticles to improve blood
flow before rinsing off.

**To enrich the nails**
Almond oil containing vitamin E
is very nutritious for the nails. You'll
hardly need an – a couple of drops
will do both hands. Rub in gently
whenever you need it.

STAR TIP
If your nails have
a slight yellow stain
from using dark-
coloured varnish,
soak your fingers or
toes in a bowl of warm
water with lemon and
lime slices, and the
stains will disappear.

# Falsies

Kim says: 'I haven't the prettiest hands in the world but I like my nails to look feminine, with long nails and nice jewellery. I have my own nails, but I have a layer of gel applied over the top to add strength so they're protected when I'm cleaning. False nails are the perfect cover-up for nail-biters but they take a lot of maintaining. My fingernails grow fast, so every 10 days or so there's a gap at the bottom. If you leave it, the nail will get top heavy and break. So you have to go back for a top up. If you want the nails removed, it's back to the salon again.'

Choose a reputable nail salon: some cheaper treatments use an adhesive called MMA (methyl methacrylate) which can damage the nail plate. Ask for EMA (ethyl methacrylate) instead.

Fungi can thrive in the moist, dark space between real and artificial nails. Look out for green or yellow discoloration, spongy nails and thick skin around the nail bed. See your GP if you're worried.

Give your nails an occasional rest. Some people say you shouldn't wear false nails for longer than a few weeks at a time.

Falsies weaken the natural nails below, so give them a nice oily treatment in between.

Clean carefully under nails with a nail-brush, soap and water, but be careful not to lift the false nail from your nail plate.

**APPLIANCE OF SCIENCE**
Long nails and false nails harbour more bacteria and fungi than short nails. This can cause nasty infections and fungal colonisation which can weaken nails permanently.

# Nail-biting

Aggie says: 'I've always bitten my nails. I remember when I was a kid, I used to bite my little sister's nails too. But when I started doing close-up television work, I was so embarrassed at seeing the state of my raggedy, stubby nails that I stopped. That was 18 months ago and I haven't bitten them since. Now I do my own nails once a week to keep them nice.'

- Biting nails and surrounding skin can damage the nails and cuticles, and cause secondary bacterial infection.

- Nearly half of teenagers bite their nails. Hypnotherapy can help with chronic nail-biting.

- Applying foul-tasting anti-biting paint can help as well (although some nail nibblers get used to the taste!), but quite frankly it's willpower that will make you stop.

# For strong nails

- Use rubber gloves when you're washing up or cleaning, and thick, protective gardening gloves when you're doing the weeding.

- If you use a keyboard, press the keys with the pads of your fingers, not your nail tips.

- Don't open breakfast cereals and other packages with your nails. So convenient, we know, but it breaks nails and lacerates fingers too.

- Tempting though it is, remember your nail is not to be used as a screwdriver or a toothpick.

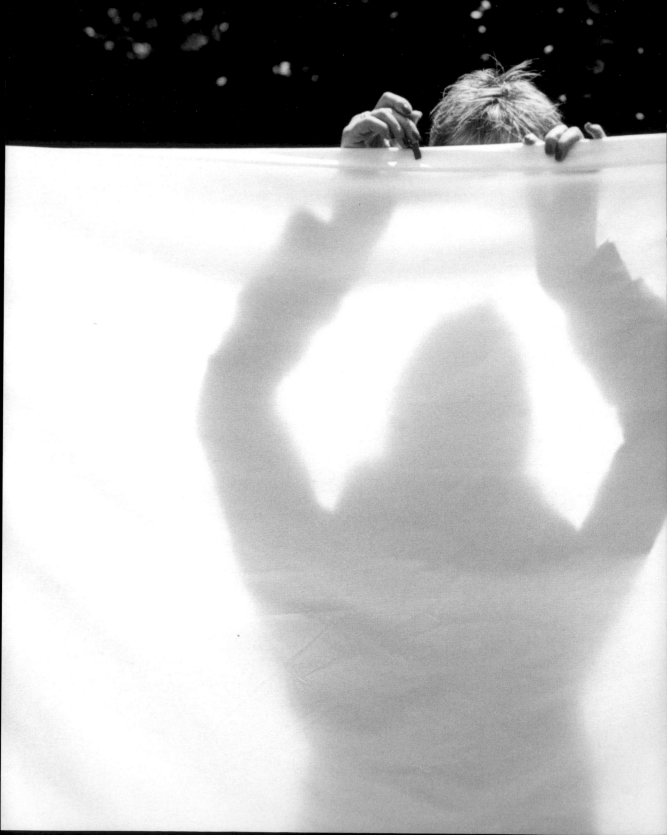

HOME LAUNDRY

Some of the bedrooms we've been in! We've had to tiptoe through the stinking, festering clothes littering the floor, in fear of catching something nasty. Some filthy so-and-so's kick weeks' worth of grey, malodorous, unwashed underwear under the bed, and just drop their crusty socks and sweaty T-shirts on the floor when they undress.

As for having a laundry method – forget it! The filthy beggars wait until they've nothing left to wear then rifle through their heaps of stinking clothes to find the underpants that haven't already got up and walked away of their own accord. Well, there's no excuse for it. Nobody should be walking round with filth all over them, not when there's a launderette on every corner and washing powders that work miracles.

Washing is awfully simple. Just get a system going. Read that label. Don't bung everything in together or it will all come out grey and lifeless.

It's important that things look good. If you look after your clothes they last longer which saves you money. And there's a wonderful satisfaction in knowing your clothes are bright and clean.

Walking round looking grubby and smelling like a damp dog? Behave yourselves. There's just no excuse for shoddy laundering – it's sheer couldn't-care-less and laziness. So get on with it. Startle yourself and put a wash on, you mucky pups.

# Do your washing regularly, or it's a heck of a battle to get things clean.

# Why washing works

Hot water is marvellous stuff. By itself it's a mild cleanser, but add in some detergent, agitate it around and you've got all the ingredients of a top class wash that will kill dirt, grease, mites, bugs and other nasties. Your clothes will look clean and sparkling and they'll smell as fresh as a daisy. Irresistible!

# Temperature control

Always read the care label inside your clothes before you wash them the first time! Then remember there are only four basic machine cycles.

○ Very hot wash is at 95°C: use this only for white cottons and linens.

○ Hot wash is at 60°C: use for coloured cottons, nappies, coloured towels and bedding – this temperature kills dust mites and gets rid of their allergens.

○ Warm wash is at 40°C: use for dark coloureds, colourfast brights and most synthetics.

○ Cool wash is at 30°C: use this for delicates and for fabrics that run or bleed.

# Washing powders and detergents

We're jolly lucky today! We have washing products for everything under the sun. In our mothers' day, all they had was a bar of green Fairy soap to rub over the clothes – the same one they used for scrubbing the floors.

Nowadays you could go mad with all the bleaches, enzymes, optical brighteners and other clothes washing treatments that are stacked on our supermarket shelves. But keep it simple. We love a biological powder for whites. The enzymes kill the stains from grass, mud, chocolate, blood, perspiration and other stinky body bits. And it's good for whitening too.

You can also buy special powders to brighten dark colours and they work a treat. Just read the labels on the packets and find something that suits you.

In hard water areas, you'll need to use more detergent and perhaps a water softener to get your wash properly clean. You can add half a cup of borax (from the pharmacy) or washing soda into the wash along with your normal detergent or use one of the proprietary water softeners on the market. Some detergents contain water softeners too.

Add fabric conditioner separately. Products that promise to clean and condition in one don't wash very well in our experience.

# Sorting the laundry

If you're one of those daft beggars who chucks the whole lot in together, no wonder your clothes look tired and grey. Sort your clothes out first. It's the secret to a good wash.

Empty pockets of dirty tissues and other detritus. Close zips and hooks so they don't catch or snag other clothes.

Check for stains. Given a pre-wash rub with soap or a stain remover, many stains will then come out without fuss in the washing machine.

Sort clothes into four piles: whites, light coloureds, dark coloureds and delicates.

*Whites* are cottons and linens, including basic white T-shirts, underwear, pillowcases and sheets that can take a hot wash at 60 or 95°C.

*Light coloureds* are pastels, patterns and those whites you don't know what to do with – the white T-shirts with coloured logos or patterns that might run, for example. These can be washed at 40 to 60°C, depending on the material.

*Dark coloureds* are dark shirts, dark underwear, socks, trousers and jeans. These go on a 40°C wash. One complication: new darks often bleed badly, so run a bowl of cold water, add loads of salt and throw the clothing in. This will prevent bleeding, but it's still best to wash on their own for the first couple of washes.

*Delicates* are woollen jumpers and blankets, fine cotton knits, embroidered items, and silk. Some wool can be machine washed (check the label) on a cool wash with a gentle spin. But it's often best to hand-wash or dry-clean delicates instead.

You're not finished yet, you know! Now put to one side clothes that produce lint – towels, towelling bathrobes etc. These should be put in a separate wash from materials such as corduroy, velvet, polyester and acrylic, which attract lint.

**STAR TIP**
There are so many different synthetic materials nowadays and, wouldn't you know it, they all have different washing needs. Check the care label before washing or you risk shrinkage and bleeding colours.

# Laundry baskets

Oh the festering clothes we've seen piled at the foot of unmade beds. For goodness sake, get a laundry basket – it makes life so much easier. Ideally you'd have three: one for whites, one for coloureds and one for delicates. But who's got room for that? One will do the job. If you're too mean to spend money on a nice cloth or wicker basket you can hang an old pillowcase on the back of your bedroom door. Anything to get that dirty linen out of sight.

Then get yourself an in-and-out system going. Dirty clothes in the laundry basket, washed clothes in the ironing basket. Not exactly complicated, now is it?

**1** The best laundry baskets are those that let air circulate. There are some lovely cotton ones on the market, or old-fashioned wicker baskets and hampers are perfect.

**2** Dry used towels and other damp items before putting them in the laundry basket, or tie damp towels in a plastic bag before you put them inside the basket. Damp clothes stink and mildew discolours fabrics, so don't let them take hold in your laundry basket.

**3** Keep your laundry basket in the bedroom rather than the bathroom. It's more convenient and stops clothes getting damp.

**4** Get right down to the bottom of your laundry basket once a week. Textile beetles and moths, which feed on human detritus, can colonise there.

**5** When clothes are washed and dry, put them in an ironing basket. We like a big white plastic one – you can buy squishy ones with handles that fit into small cupboards, but anything that lets air circulate through nicely will do.

**6** To keep laundry baskets fresh, sprinkle baking powder or bicarbonate of soda into the laundry bag once or twice a week to freshen things up nicely. Fine if it goes in the machine when you come round to washing the clothes.

**APPLIANCE OF SCIENCE**
One of the honkers we swabbed had as much bacteria on the clothes in his 'clean' laundry bag as he did in the 'dirty' laundry bag. His trick was to put washed but damp clothes in a plastic bag where they festered nicely. Make sure your clothes air after washing, then put them away.

# How to machine wash

Aren't we the lucky ones to have machines to wash our clothes for us? A generation ago, wash day was a dreadful drudge and no mistake. It took the whole day. On a Monday, those poor women had to boil the water, scrub the clothes on the washboard, then rinse and mangle the excess water out of them. It was hot and heavy work. Now we just pop our clothes in the washing machine and they come out fresh and sparkling an hour later. We don't know we're born!

For the freshest clothes, you need to get a machine wash routine going. You'll soon get the hang of it, and it'll become second nature.

**1** After sorting clothes, pre-treat stains by rubbing a proprietary stain remover or a little liquid detergent into grubby areas. Cuffs and collars are quick to pick up bodily oils and grease.

**2** Turn corduroy, velvet and any clothes that pill (bobble), inside out.

**3** Place clothes in the machine and check you haven't overloaded it. If you're washing synthetics, don't fill the machine quite as full. Synthetics need more space and water because when they rub against each other they cause pills – those little fabric balls – to form.

**4** Choose your cycle. Modern washing machines are wonderful inventions. You can choose cold rinses and short spins for more delicate or synthetic fabrics if you wish.

**5** Remember to use the pre-wash cycle if your clothes look as though you've been rolling around in a muddy field.

**6** Add your detergent and fabric conditioner (if using) in the drawer dispenser. Or put tablets in the drum following the manufacturer's instructions. Don't forget to switch on the machine.

**7** When the load is finished, take clothes out and hang them to dry. If you leave wet clothes in the drum, they'll start to smell.

**APPLIANCE OF SCIENCE**
Washing socks at 60°C with detergent will kill off the fungus that causes athlete's foot.

# How to hand wash

Doing a good hand wash is wonderfully soothing, rather like making bread. Use rubber gloves if your hands are sensitive. It's good for all delicates, wool and underwear. It's fine to use soap if you don't have any gentle detergent.

1. Fill a basin with warm water. Add a splash of mild, hand-washing detergent.

2. Put your clothes in the basin and leave them to soak for a few minutes.

3. Then start lifting and kneading them gently. This helps the detergent to extract grime and grease.

4. If clothes are badly stained, leave to soak for half an hour, then come back and knead gently again.

5. Pull out the plug and drain the soapy water away.

6. Fill up the basin with clean, lukewarm water and rinse clothes well. Rinse until the water is clear to get rid of all traces of detergent.

7. Gently squeeze out clothes. Hardier garments can be given a short spin cycle in the machine. Otherwise, roll clothes in a towel and stamp on them. Reshape garments, then hang out or lay flat to dry.

# Traveller's tricks

If you need a T-shirt for next morning, rub the smelly bits – usually the collar and armpits – with bar soap, then wash the rest of it and rinse in cold water. Wring out, then place flat on a towel. Roll up the towel like a sausage and stamp on it so the towel absorbs the moisture. Hang the T-shirt on a hanger overnight. It should be dry in the morning and there's no need to iron it.

**STAR TIP**
Hang stinky socks out of the window. UV rays kill off many bacteria.

# How to wash whiter and brighter

Dingy grey clothes are not what we want to see. If your laundry is looking tired and wizened, try these sparkling tricks.

○ With white cotton, add a large glass of clear distilled vinegar to the rinse cycle. The acetic acid brightens up white clothes.

○ Clothes sometimes come out grey because the washing machine is overloaded. Soiled clothes don't get properly clean so don't overfill.

○ Add a cupful of borax to the wash. It acts as a colour booster.

○ Bleach can work – but only on whites, and never use it on synthetics. Add a cupful to a bucket of water, soak clothes for half an hour, rinse, then wash as normal. Test for bleach fastness first if you're worried.

○ Net curtain whitener is good and powerful, even for synthetics. Leave whites to soak in it for five minutes or add it to the washing machine cycle.

# To get dazzling white sheets

Run a bath with hot, hot water and add a generous amount of biological washing powder. Open a window, for heaven's sake, you don't want everything steaming up. Leave the sheets in the bath for eight hours or overnight. Next morning rinse and wring them out, or put them through a wash. They will be beautiful. This is two in one, because when you pull the plug out your bath will be spotless and smiling at you, too.

# How to wash silk

We always hand wash silk. The label says dry-clean only, but in some dry-cleaners it can cost £5 to do a silk tie. Die a pauper if you want, dear, or learn to wash properly. People are lousy washers – they can't be bothered. So take your time or don't bother.

You can buy a bottle of silk wash but, honestly, toilet soap will do. Take your blouse or tie and gently immerse it in cold water. Rub a bit of soap over it and softly squeeze it between the fingers. Rinse in cold water. Put in a bit of softener, and rinse again.

Then put a light coloured towel on the floor and place your washed garment on it. If it's a blouse, put the buttons together and spread the sleeves out. Roll it up in the towel like a sausage, then stamp on it. That's it, washed.

Whip it out, shake, shake, shake, and put it on a hanger to dry. If you're ironing it later, be cautious. Use a cool iron and put a bit of brown paper or white tissue paper over it. Don't press the iron hard – be like a fairy going over it. All done? Lovely, isn't it!

Kim says 'If I'm out somewhere and the sun's beating down, I'll take a spare pair of briefs and pop them on. Goodness, do I feel fresher.'

# How often to change and wash undies

You have to change your knickers every day, and twice a day in the heat when your bra and briefs stick to your bits. Let's be blunt, while they're sticking to you they're working their way up your bum and there's nothing more uncomfortable.

As for bras, well! Some of the mucky pups we met on our travels had worn the same bra for months on end. The straps were stiff with muck and they were showing them off to the world. It was horrible! If you want to flash your straps make sure they're clean first, will you?

You've got to change your bra every day. Let's face it, under the arms and across the ribs, perspiration hits hard and that elastic and bone can get very mucky. Don't be disgraceful. How big are these things to wash?

# Kim's way to wash undies

Whenever I get in, I half-fill a plastic bowl with a teacup of biological washing powder and water. I drop my briefs and bra in as soon as I take them off. Sometimes I wash them that evening, sometimes I leave them till next morning. I rinse them by running them under a cold tap and they are sparkling! Occasionally I put briefs in the machine, but I truly think lingerie should go in a bowl with a bit of biological. I can't help myself, I just do.

## To clean grubby bras

Take any bar of toilet soap, wet it and rub along the straps and mucky bits of the bra. Then you can drop the bra – light colours only mind, not dark – into the bowl with the biological. You can leave them in there for two or three days until they're ice cold. They come out so bright they're smiling at you.

If you want to wash bras in the machine, buy a mesh zip up bag, stick four or five bras in there and put them on a delicate cycle. Don't put a bra or girdle in the dryer or it'll last you a third of the time. They contain a good deal of elastic and the heat destroys it. What a waste of good money!

**STAR TIP**
70 per cent of women wear the wrong size bra – which affects posture, shape and can harm your health. Get fitted in a specialist bra shop or department store.

# To whiten a bra

Use a product for whitening net curtains. After washing, put a sachet into a bowl of cold water (not hot, it will perish the elastic) and immerse the bra overnight. Rinse.

# To have sweet-smelling underwear

Using fabric conditioner with undies softens the elastic. Instead, take your favourite perfume or cologne, spritz a bit of it into the last rinse and swill around. They'll have a lovely fragrance!

# Allergy prevention

If you get the itches, change your brand of washing powder to an eco-friendly one and make sure you rinse clothes well to get rid of all traces of detergent. Do hot washes, where possible, rather than cold. Dust mites are only killed off at temperatures of 60°C and over. At the very least, hot wash your bed linen once a week, and your mattress cover as often as possible. Mites can live in clothes too, so hot wash these whenever you can.

**APPLIANCE OF SCIENCE**
After a day's wear, a bra will normally contain around 1,000 bacteria. We took swabs from one poor soul's bra and found it was saturated with 80 million bacteria crawling all over it, putting her at risk of nasty skin lesions and infections.

# Laundry blunders

There should be a compulsory government scheme to teach people how to do laundry. It would save people a lot of money buying new clothes if they didn't make these blunders.

### Chucking everything in together

If you stuff the machine with blacks, whites and pinks then it'll come out with not a white thing that isn't grey, and not a black thing that hasn't had the life bled out of it. Wash by colour and don't wash blacks in hot water.

### Overfilling the washing machine

If you load up your washing machine until you need a boot to get the rest in, it's too full. People say, oh I can't be bothered doing two or three washes, let's get it all in one. But at the end you've got the dirtiest, greyest washing. There needs to be enough room for the water and detergent to get round and agitate nicely.

### Bleeding into the rest of the wash

If this happens to you, don't dry the load. Instead, remove the offending article and rewash the rest of the clothes immediately using the hottest water the load will take.

### Pilling and bobbling

To prevent pilling, turn garments inside out before washing or put them in a mesh bag. Try a gentler, shorter spin cycle as well.

### Over drying

This frizzles, shrinks and yellows clothes. Don't dry clothes until they're bone dry. Ironing and airing will take care of the rest.

# What needs dry-cleaning?

A lot of clothes that say 'dry-clean only' on the label can be hand-washed and come up beautifully. But you need washing skills – and we do call them skills! Most importantly, you've got to know your fibre. To test it out, go to a material shop and buy the smallest amount you can of the same fabric. Then cut it into four and do all sorts with it: put one in very hot water, another in warm water, one in cold water or try out different detergents – see which comes out best. It costs you 50p to learn that, and you'll save pounds on dry-cleaning bills.

Still, we always take pure wool skirts and very delicate fabrics to the dry-cleaners. In some cases, it's safer.

## Spot cleaning

Good for dark wool skirts or trousers or anything that needs dry cleaning. Put the dirty item over the ironing board, take a wet cotton hankie or face flannel and gently rub away any marks on the material. Then press. If using a good steam iron, you can hold it half an inch away and steam without the iron touching the fabric. This stops you getting a shine on the fabric.

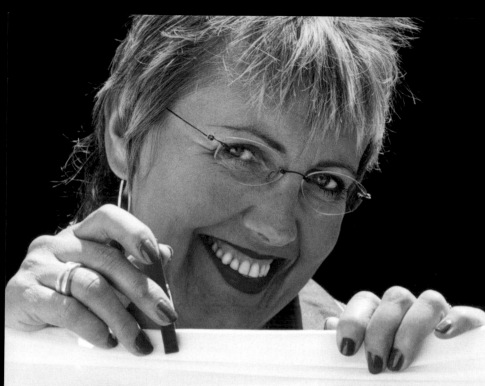

# Blow those clothes dry

Aggie says: 'What could be better than the smell of laundry fresh from the washing line, after a day blowing in a balmy breeze? There's a lovely freshness about it which can't be beaten. Whenever possible, Kim and I are out there with the pegs, gamely battling the elements. But in winter, it's another story. We still like to air dry clothes rather than using a tumble dryer. Here's how to maximise your drying potential.'

Hang as many items as you can on coat hangers. Hang these along a sturdy shower rail or a clothes horse. Leave enough space between items for them to dry.

Move your clothes horse around the house. Standing it near radiators, air vents or a fan will help speed things up. You can buy retractable clothes lines to put up over the bath.

When stacking a clothes horse, use every inch of space but don't overlap clothes or they won't dry. Put small items like pants and socks at the bottom, and work up to larger, heavier items like trousers and towels at the top.

# Using a tumble dryer

Clothes – especially synthetics – shrink terribly in a tumble dryer. They get a real beating from the agitation and harsh heat. Knicker elastic goes twangy and you get nasty pills all over your tops. So, if you have to use a dryer, use it with caution.

**1** First check there's no lint in the dryer and clean out the lint filter to stop those annoying white bits of fluff getting all over your clean clothes.

**2** Don't put delicates, knits or drip dry clothes in the dryer. Hang them out or dry them flat instead.

**3** Choose the drying cycle you want. Sort by material. Synthetics don't take long to dry and need a lower temperature. Heavy cottons like towels and jeans take longer to dry and can go on full temperature.

**4** Shake out clothes before you place them in the tumble dryer to get rid of creases.

**5** If you overload the dryer you just get a wodge of soggy clothes an hour later. Leave enough space in the drum for air to get all around the clothes.

**6** Check synthetics after 15 minutes. Better to finish them off near a radiator or vent than fry them in the tumble dryer.

**7** Check all clothes after 30 minutes. Take out those that are nearly dry. They'll shrink and turn yellow if you leave them in. We like to finish them off with an iron and an air rather than letting them get so bone dry they can stand up by themselves.

**8** Fold or hang clothes as you take them out of the dryer.

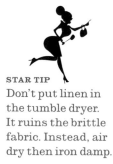

**STAR TIP**
Don't put linen in the tumble dryer. It ruins the brittle fabric. Instead, air dry then iron damp.

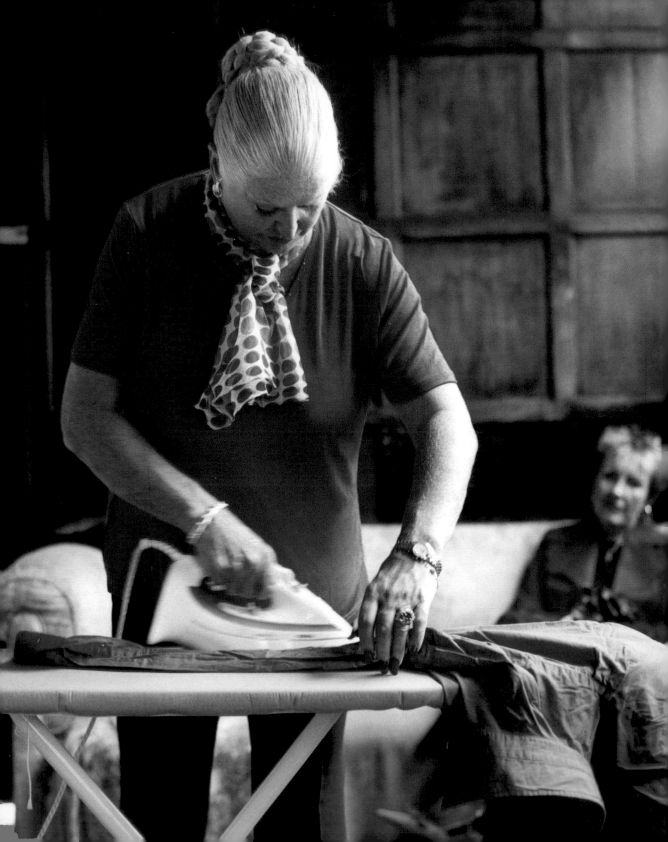

# Ironing

Here's the gospel according to Kim.

You often hear people saying they don't iron and are proud of it. Well, dear, fine if you want to go round looking like a ragbag. But not me, thank you very much!

If you wash, you've got to iron. It's terribly essential. I can't say I love it, but it has to be done, and best if you can whisk through it quickly. Paying a bit more for a good steam iron with a large water trough will make the job speedier – no use if you have to keep filling up every minute.

Ideally you should wash and iron the same day or the next day. If you leave it, please don't let it go for more than a week or you'll have a pile six feet high and nobody can face that. Besides, who's got enough clothes to last that long?

The secret to easy ironing is to iron clothes a bit damp. If they're bone dry, they're a beggar to get through. But not fully damp, mind, just so the cloth has a bit of coldness about it. I hold it to my cheek and that tells you when it's right. Then you can whizz through the ironing like a dose of salts. After it's done, hang clothes out on a clothes horse in a warm room to air. Next morning, they'll be perfect!

# Whizz through the ironing
## like a dose of salts.

### To make a pressing cloth

Go and buy a cotton pillowcase – but don't pay a lot for it. Undo the seams and open it out. There, you have a wonderful pressing cloth that will protect clothes from scorch and shine!

### To avoid shine

Iron on the wrong side or use a pressing cloth.

### To declog your steam iron

No need to buy expensive descalers. Instead, pour some clear distilled vinegar into the water tank, turn the iron on, and allow to steam for several minutes. Then cool the iron and rinse through with cold water.

### To iron a cotton sheet

You need a good steam iron for this. Fold your sheet in half, then in half again. That way it won't drag over the floor. Put it on the ironing board, then full steam ahead all over it. With a powerful iron the steam will go right through the sheet. Turn it over and do it again. Hang out to air. Now how quick was that?

### To iron a shirt sleeve

Kim says: 'I never use shirt ironing boards. Too fiddly by half. Shirts are easy to do if you don't mind a crease in the sleeve, but if you don't want a crease, here's how to do it. Iron the cuffs first. Then put the sleeve on the ironing board with the seam at one side. Iron up to the top of the sleeve. Turn and do the other side. Because the iron is narrower than the sleeve, you won't put a crease in the edges. Then turn the sleeve so the seam is facing you in the middle, and iron up to the top. There, a crease-free sleeve in seconds!'

### Don't bother ironing . . .

Underwear, towels, nappies, velvet or any material with a nap.

**APPLIANCE OF SCIENCE**
Ironing with a soleplate temperature between 110 and 200°C (one to three stars on ironing guides) kills most remaining micro-organisms in the material left after washing.

# Out, darned spot!

You need to move fast with stains. Don't be sitting around chatting while it's drying – get to it as quick as you can and start dabbing.

Kim always carries a white cotton hankie with her for spills. 'I don't like tissues because they break up. When I tip something down myself, I get to the loo quickly, dip my hankie in water and rub on some ordinary toilet soap. Then I get my hand inside my blouse, and dab away at the stain. Even if it doesn't fade completely, I'll have killed and diluted 80 per cent of it. I swear by my white cotton hankie with finger and toilet soap. It is marvellous, just marvellous!'

You can buy those fancy stain removers, but in most cases, good old-fashioned household products like clear distilled vinegar, white toothpaste, baking soda, bleach and soap work wonders – although never all together, or the fumes will knock you for six and you'll ruin the garment. Work from the back of the stain and push it forward and out if you can. An old toothbrush is good on stubborn, dried stains, but don't go rubbing away on delicate fabrics or the garment will end up in shreds. Remember, heat can set a stain, so don't use hot water or iron over it.

With stains, be gentle and persistent. Keep rubbing and blotting, rubbing and blotting, and any stain will come out a treat.

### Antiperspirant and deodorant stains

Tricky if they're old and caked on. Try tepid water and toilet soap first. If the stain is still there, soak in a weak solution of clear distilled vinegar and baking soda (test on a bit of the material where it won't be seen to make sure it won't damage the material). Rinse, then wash.

### Blood

Move fast here. Rinse the garment in cold – not hot – water. People always say use salt but we apply biological washing detergent or use a bar of soap to gently massage out the stain. If the stain remains in white fabric, use bleach. For dried bloodstains, soak overnight in a bucket of water with some biological washing powder. Works miracles!

### Candlewax

Scrape off as much as you can. Put paper towels or brown paper under and over the stain. Press with a warm iron – the paper will absorb the melted wax.

### Chewing gum

Fold your garment up, place it in a plastic bag, and leave it in the freezer overnight. The next day, the gum will ping off easily! If any bits remain, take a pair of tweezers and pick them out. Always use a plastic bag or the cloth will stick to everything else in the freezer and you'll tear it to shreds when you take it out.

### Chocolate

Scrape off as much as possible, wet the stain, then gently rub in some liquid biological detergent or good quality concentrated washing-up liquid. Wash as normal.

### Coffee, tea, wine and other alcoholic drinks

These are easier than you think if you act quickly. Dab the stain with soda water, keep blotting off, putting on, blotting off with white paper towels. Always keep a bottle of soda water in your house – it is wonderful with red wine stains. If you get a water mark, take a white face cloth or tea towel, put it under the tap, wring it out, put it over the water mark and stamp on it with your feet for a few seconds, then wash as usual.

## Grass

Put a load of white toothpaste on the stain and rub until the whole area is covered. Leave for a few hours. When you go back, put your hand under the stain and rub a bit of soap over the toothpaste under warm running water. The stain will be out!

## Grease, butter and oil

Try soaking in washing-up liquid and warm water, or dampen the fabric and rub with toilet soap. If the material is fragile, give in and buy a proprietary stain remover for greasy stains.

## Ink

Ballpoint pens are a curse, leaking all over pockets and clothes. Hair spray works a treat. Spray on, allow to dry, then wash as normal.

## Ketchup and tomato products

You can remove this with men's shaving cream. Just a tiny marble-sized ball in the palm of your hand will do. Using your finger, gently massage it in. Patience pays off here – it might take 10 minutes.

## Make-up and lipstick

Most make-up comes off easily. Rub some toilet soap into the stain, leave for 30 minutes, then wash out. Waterproof mascara is harder. Soak the stained bit in a teacup with biological powder or washing-up liquid then wash as normal.

## Mildew

Outside, remove as much mildew as you can with a soft brush. Use a mix of bleach and water, following the instructions. If there's mildew on the shower curtain, rub with toilet soap, washing-up liquid, or vinegar and put in the washing machine on a cold wash.

## Mud

The secret is to leave mud to dry – then it comes off with no problem. Just brush excess off and launder as normal.

## Perspiration

Sponge fresh perspiration stains with a solution of ammonia, if the fabric allows, following the instructions on the bottle. Old stains can be soaked in a little clear distilled vinegar and water. Then wash as normal and they'll come out a treat.

## Ring around the collar and cuffs

This is caused by body oils. To keep shirts fresh, rub toilet soap gently over the soiled areas and then wash as normal.

## DISCLAIMER

All the natural mixes are tried and tested. Never mix commercial cleaning products as the combination can create toxic fumes. Never mix bleach or ammonia with any other products.

**STAR TIP**

Always have some denture cleaning tablets – the ones that fizz – in the house. They take out stains wonderfully in light coloured clothes. Dilute a couple in a bowl with warm water then leave your stained clothing in overnight. Works well on tea, coffee, smoke, grapefruit, blackcurrant and other colourful stains.

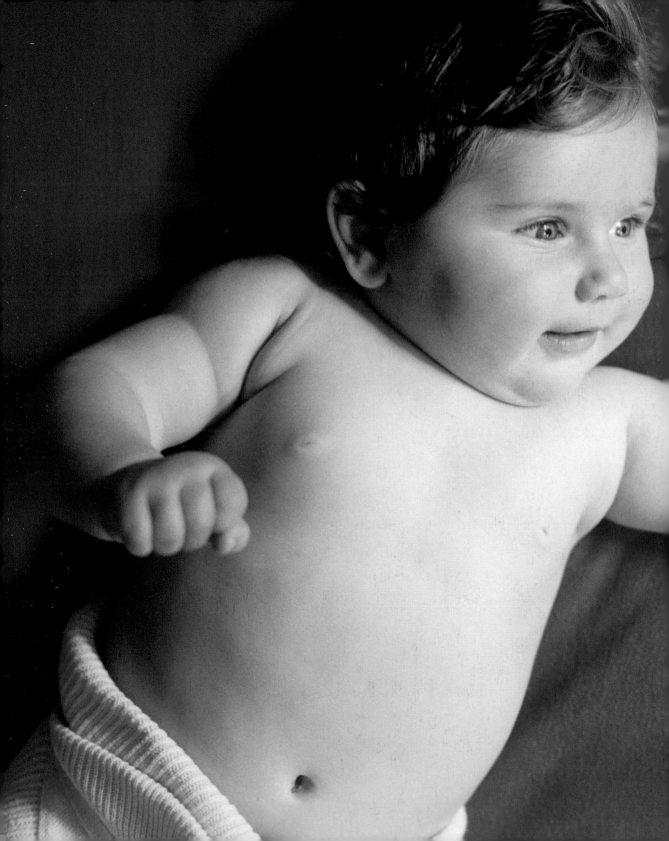

# Washing nappies

Aggie says: 'You're doing the environment a favour if you can avoid using disposables. For ease, use a nappy service if there's one in your area, although washing nappies yourself is not the chore you might think.'

1 With cloth nappies at least you get rid of the poo immediately. Scrape off excess and flush it down the loo.

2 Put soiled nappies in a bucket with a lid with a handful of borax and some chlorine bleach to deodorise and remove stains. Or buy special nappy soaking products.

3 Wash nappies at 60°C in a separate wash every couple of days.

4 Only put about a dozen nappies maximum into your machine at once. Over packing the machine means they just won't wash properly.

5 Don't use fabric conditioner – it makes nappies less absorbent.

6 There's no need to waste your time ironing nappies. Just air, fold and put them away.

**STAR TIP**
After you've changed a nappy, don't wash your hands in the kitchen sink, because it can spread faecal matter into the food production chain and contaminate the kitchen taps. Always use the washbasin in the loo instead.

# Gym etiquette

After you've been to the gym and had a shower, don't spoil it all by putting your sweat-stained pants or knickers and bra back on. Treat yourself to some fresh, clean ones.

Wash your sweaty sports gear at soon as possible. If you're not doing a wash for a few days, don't let it fester. Dry out gym gear naturally before chucking it in the laundry basket or it will stink the place out.

# Jewels and gems

Yes, these are grubby, too, wouldn't you know it. If you don't believe us, take off your watch and smell the back of the strap – ugh! Bacteria hides in all those little crevices. Buy a new leather strap at least once a year and buff it up regularly with some leather cleaner so it doesn't pong.

**To clean silver jewellery**
Line a small bowl with silver foil, shiny side up, and fill with warm water. Pour in a handful of soda crystals and let them dilute. Put your silver jewellery in the water and soak for a few minutes. Rinse and buff gently with a clean cloth.

**To clean under rings**
Around one of our minger's rings we found massive amounts of bacteria including *staphylococcus aureus* which can cause nasty skin infections. If you can't get rings off, clean under them with a pair of tweezers and antibacterial wipes.

**To clean gold jewellery**
Drop it into a glass of cola and leave to soak for a few minutes. Rinse and buff up with a soft cloth.

**Body piercings**
These sites – especially tummy, tongue and outer ear – can get infected easily. Mouth piercings are particularly dangerous, increasing the risk of serious bacterial and viral infections. Keep jewellery clean, swab the site with saline solution when needed, and brush tongue jewellery every time you clean your teeth to stop plaque forming.

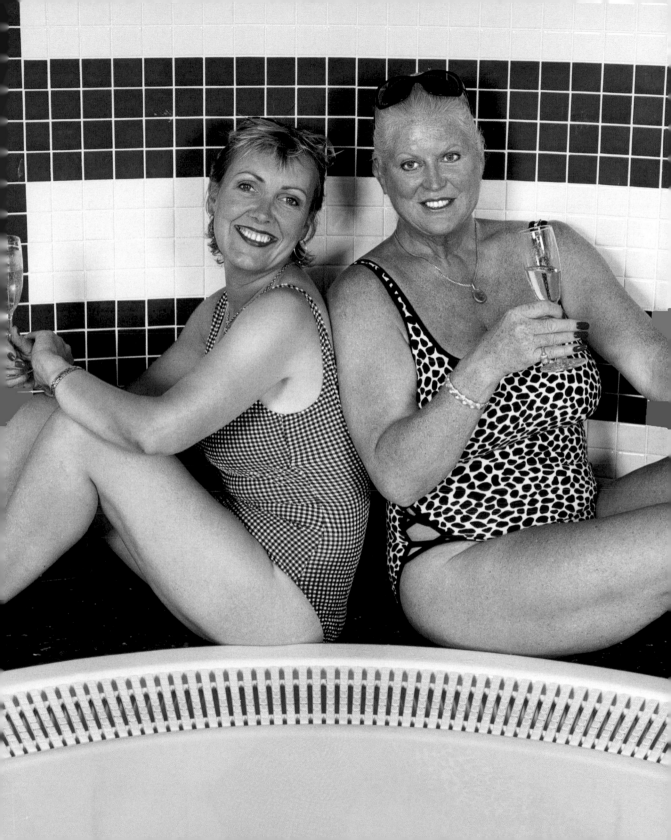

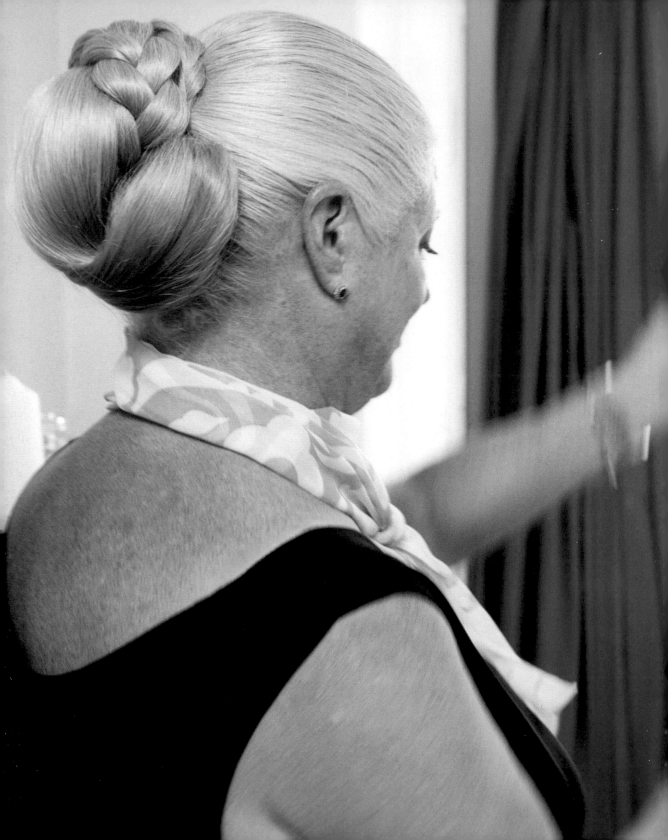

# THE LIVING
ENVIRONMENT

We've seen some heinous home hygiene in our mission to tame those unlawful soap-dodgers. Ooh, the bedrooms of some of these stinking soap-dodgers stank to high heaven. Filthy! If you're going to be a clean person, you need a clean home, too. You can't just emerge spotless from a stinking hell hole. If your bed is full of muck and bugs, and your bath is coated in grease, grime and hair, you can't expect to get yourself properly clean.

The bedroom and bathroom are private spaces. We spend more time in them than any other rooms in the house. It's where we go to strip off and relax, not drown and choke in a sea of clutter and dust. We all want sweet dreams in the bedroom – and if we're lucky some nights of rip-roaring passion.

So banish your clutter, keep the dust down, and open some windows. It really is that simple. In a clean, healthy, bedroom you'll sleep soundly, dream fondly and emerge each morning as fresh as a daisy!

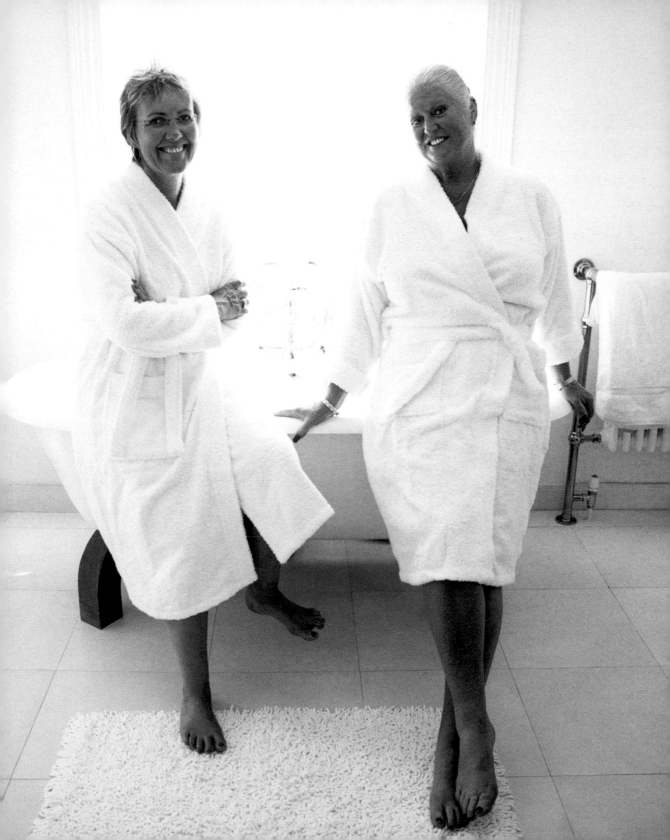

# Keep your bedroom clean

The bedroom is a dust bucket, yet we spend most of our home lives in there snoring, snorting and snuffling it all up. A lungful of dust is never a good thing. Dust contains dead skin, bacterial micro-organisms, pet dander, mould, dust mites and their faeces. No wonder it gets right up our noses and causes allergic reactions and asthma. To make your nights more comfortable, give the bedroom a good, weekly dust-up. And don't swish it, lift it.

## Once a week:

○ Dust the room and vacuum the carpet, including along the edges of the skirting board where dirt piles up.

○ Pull out the bed and give it a good vacuum underneath. If you store things under your bed, make it easy for yourself by using storage boxes that slide out.

○ Dust behind your radiator. If this is too narrow for the smallest vacuum cleaner nozzle, tie a damp rag around a garden stick. It even gets between double radiators.

○ Dust your blinds. Use the upholstery tool on the vacuum cleaner for roman blinds. Slatted blinds are a nightmare to clean with a duster. Instead, put on a pair of white cotton disposable gloves and run your fingers along each slat.

○ Shake out and vacuum your curtains. Vacuum up the dust bunnies that lurk on top of the wardrobe. We prefer not to store things on top of the wardrobe. But if you have to, make sure they get a weekly once-over to prevent dust becoming airborne.

**STAR TIP**
If you're buying bedroom carpet for an old house, don't go for beige. In Victorian houses the carpet bordering the skirting board often turns black because of porous bricks. It's virtually impossible to get the stain out.

# Dilute the dust

Ventilation is the secret to controlling dust and dust mites. They love a warm, humid room, full of dust and dander. We each perspire about half a pint of sweat into our beds and bedroom air each night. This damp environment and the heat from our warm bodies turns our beds into dust mite heaven – did you know a bed can contain up to two million of the little monsters? You'll never get rid of them all unless you move to the Sahara desert. But you can control them. Circulate the air, air the bed, and you'll halt the armies of dust mites in their tracks.

○ Every morning, open your bedroom window for at least an hour. Even better, open two windows to get a nice through breeze. This lowers humidity.

○ Sleep with a window slightly open at night if you can and it's safe to do so.

○ As soon as you get up in the morning, pull back the bedcovers. Let the bed air for at least an hour while you're showering and having breakfast.

○ Dust mites don't like room temperatures below 21°C. Turn down the heating in the bedroom if you suffer from dust mite allergies.

**APPLIANCE OF SCIENCE**
Inside your house, there are around 400 to 900 microbes per cubic metre of air. You inhale around 10,000 of these micro-organisms every day. These include moulds, fungi and bacteria that cause respiratory illness, nasal irritation and allergies.

# Pillows and pillowcases

Pillowcases get dirty quickly. You know we drool away all night, lovey, but that's not the worst of it. There's the grime and grease from hair, the sebum from our sweaty faces, plus other nasty incidentals like mucus, tears, blood and perspiration. No wonder pillowcases age so quickly. To stop them turning that waxy, yellowy colour they need a bit of love and attention.

○ Put pillow protectors beneath your pillowcases. They stop body oils and perspiration from reaching your pillow. Using allergen-proof covers also protects you from dust mites and their allergens.

○ Change and launder your pillowcases every few days. Do the sniff test: if they smell stale, chuck them in the machine straight away.

○ Wash pillow protectors at 60°C once a month, or more frequently if heavily soiled.

○ Soak stained pillowcases overnight in warm water and a cup of biological washing powder. Then rinse well or launder as normal.

○ Take pillows outside for a sunny day's airing once a month. Bash them hard to get the dust out!

○ If you think your feather pillow is full of dust mites, tie it in a plastic bag and put it in the freezer for six hours. This kills the dust mites, and washing will get rid of their faeces.

○ Wash pillows twice a year. Even feather pillows can be laundered. Check the label, and use a mild detergent. They need tumble drying: if your tumble dryer is not large enough, take them to the launderette. Adding a few new tennis balls to the dryer will prevent the feathers bunching together.

○ Chuck out polyester pillows when they start to bunch, and feather pillows when they get thin.

**APPLIANCE OF SCIENCE**
More dust mites live in the bedroom than in any other room in the house. In a six-year-old pillow, a tenth of the weight is likely to be skin flakes, dust mites and their droppings.

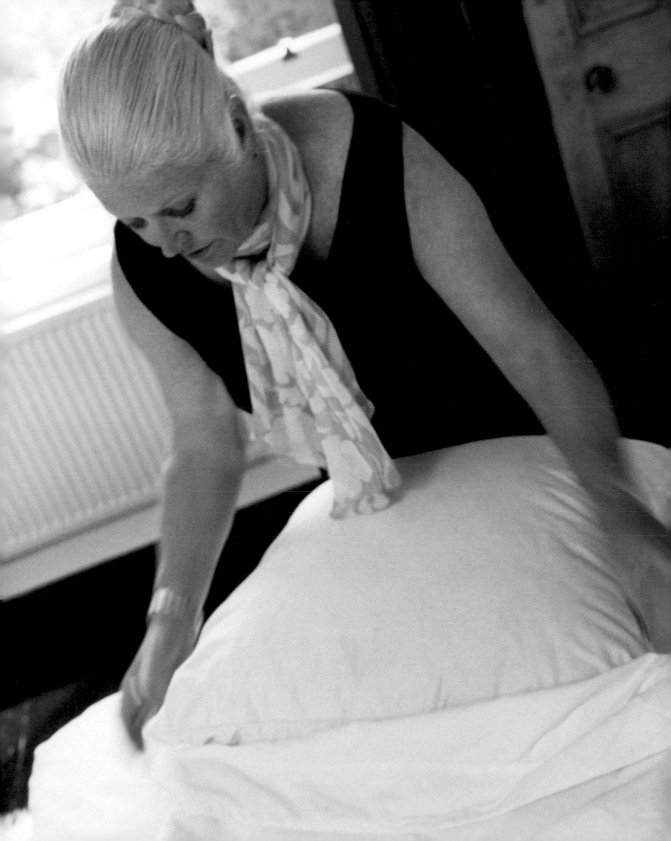

# Sheets

The human body is a marvellous thing, but doesn't some stuff come out its orifices? And there it lies, all over your sheets. Wash them! And regularly. Please, please, please don't ever go longer than nine days without a change. Be considerate, now! If we have to come and do a sniff test, we might just pass out.

○ Change sheets once a week, and in hot weather twice a week.

○ Laundering cotton sheets in 60°C kills dust mites and gets rid of their allergens. But always check the care label first.

○ Polyester sheets pill and irritate in warm weather when you perspire more. Buy cotton if you can.

○ Polyester/cotton mix sheets don't need as much attention as pure cotton. Wash in a warm cycle, but don't overload the machine. Shake them out, leave to dry, and there should be no ironing and no creases.

○ We like white cotton sheets – you know you can launder them at high temperatures. If you buy coloured sheets, make sure they are colourfast.

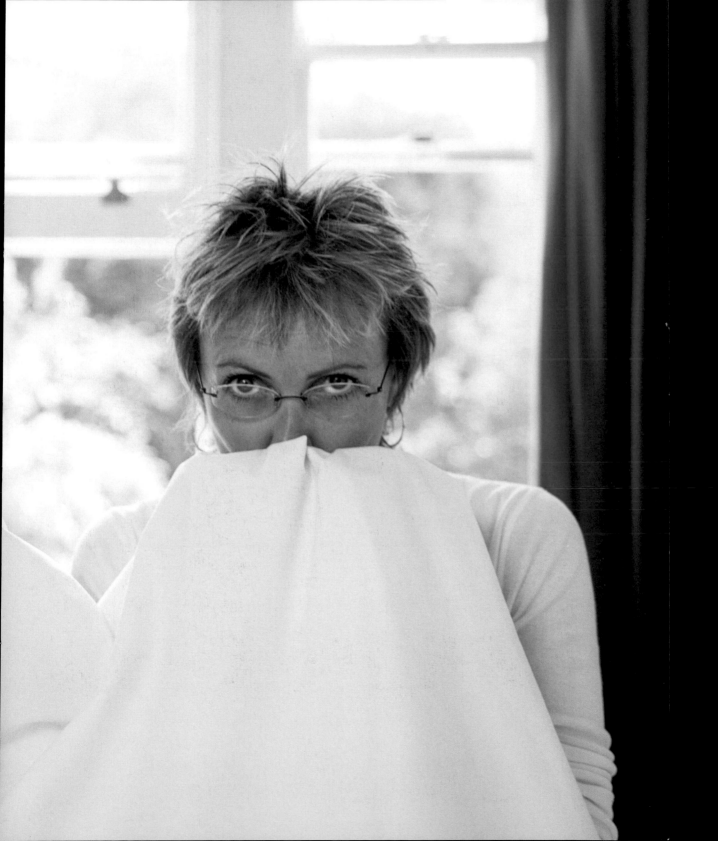

# Mattress matters

Good mattresses don't come cheap, do they now? So keep yours in peak condition by treating it to a bit of TLC.

- Use a mattress protector, and launder it once a month.

- Turn the mattress at least once a month, alternating ends or sides each time.

- If you can, take your mattress for an air outside a couple of times a year. Warm sun kills off bacteria and the airing gets rid of dust.

- Keep your mattress fresh. Vacuum it with the crevice nozzle every couple of months. To get rid of stale smells, sprinkle some bicarbonate of soda on it, leave for a couple of hours, then vacuum off.

- Don't let the kids bounce on your mattress. It ages it terribly, and shocks the bed supports into an early grave.

# Bed covers

We like a down duvet rather than blankets. And why not? They're so reasonably priced nowadays that you can even buy summer and winter weight ones. Look for a duvet that's nicely stitched together in squares, rather than in long panels. Then when you wash it, the feathers won't clump together at one end.

Some people like the weight of blankets on a bed. So long as you wash your sheets regularly, blankets only need washing once a year. Wool ones need gentle treatment so check the care label before you do any serious damage.

○ When you make the bed, put a top sheet under your duvet cover. Duvet covers aren't as hardy as sheets and what a faff it is taking them on and off! That way, your cover will stay clean longer and you'll only need to launder it once every couple of weeks.

○ Wash your duvet once or twice a year, following the care instructions. Take it to the launderette where they have big washers and dryers rather than flogging your own machine at home.

○ Put the duvet in the dryer with four new white tennis balls. The bouncing and bashing will stop the feathers bunching. If you use different duvets for summer and winter, launder them before putting away for the season.

○ Decorative cushions and throws on the bed also collect dirt and harbour dust mites. Wash or dry clean them once or twice a year.

○ Blankets and fancy bedcoverings should be laundered or dry cleaned once a year.

# What to wear in bed

Kim says: 'I like to sleep in the raw – why put clothes on to go to bed? When I was a kid, we used to have to pile on cardies to go to bed. By jove, it was so cold we even put our coats on top of the blankets. But now we've all got central heating, why bother to dress up for bed?'

Still, if you wear a nightie or pyjamas, you have to wash them regularly to get rid of the buckets of sweat we pour out each night. If you're a clean person who showers daily, then you can get away with wearing a nightie for three or four nights. Smell it. Lift it up to your nostrils and as soon as it's stale and sweaty, give it a wash.

Nighties are loose between your legs, but pyjamas press up against your nether regions. They're hitting the spot! Change pyjama trousers every day, just as you change your knickers.

# Phew, what a pong! Let's get washing, dear.

# For a wonderful wardrobe

There's nothing worse than clutter tipping out of a wardrobe that's bursting so full the doors won't close. You can get lost for weeks in there looking for a simple white blouse. You can drown and choke in all that rubbish. Get rid of it! Sort it through and chuck out the things you haven't worn for two years. You're never going to wear it again, and the charity shop will be glad of it.

Then, for heaven's sake, get yourself a system going. Sort out your summer and winter clothes and pack the out of season ones away. There! Now you've got some space in your wardrobe to get things just as you want them.

Aggie says: 'I like to keep my summer holiday clothes – shorts, swimwear and strappy, spangly things that never see the light of day at home – separate. I put them away sparkling clean in a big bag. I know exactly where they are, and can pack for holidays in two seconds flat.'

# Clothes care

Let's come clean – we all spend a small fortune on clothes, so why not treat them with a bit of love and respect.

○ Launder or dry clean out of season clothes before you put them away – dirty, sweaty fabrics are a banquet for moths. Don't iron them, though. They'll only get crumpled.

○ Invest in some wooden coat hangers with trouser and skirt clips. You needn't pay the earth for them, some large retailers sell them very cheaply.

○ For a sensible wardrobe, order your clothes from left to right, with all clothes facing the same way. Try: coats, evening wear, shirts, skirts, trousers and suits or whatever system suits you.

○ Hang cedar bark chunks on your coat hangers to discourage moths. Once or twice a year, rub them over with sandpaper to re-invigorate them.

○ Hang belts up inside the wardrobe to get them out of the way. Fit a couple of cup hooks and hang belts by the buckle.

○ Sort yourself out an underwear drawer. Put in a drawer liner first, to stop fabrics snagging on the wood. To make undies smell fresh, pop in some pot pourri, a hankie sprayed with your favourite fragrance, or little gift bars of soap, unwrapped.

○ Store fine items such as cashmere jumpers on shelves in scented, zippable plastic bags to protect them from moth larvae and mildew. Or use old pillowcases.

○ Leave clothes that have been dry cleaned inside the protective plastic bag until you wear them. It keeps the dust off. Then air before you wear. Dust builds up inside a wardrobe. Once a month, dust and vacuum inside. Your clothes will thank you for it.

# Shoes

We love our shoes but they need looking after or you have a heck of a mess at the bottom of your wardrobe. In the old days Sunday night was shoe-polishing night, to get them looking smart for a week's work or school. We still like to do ours then – but whatever suits you.

Use a fabric shoe hanger to save space. If you must keep your shoes at the bottom of the wardrobe, put your best pairs in boxes to protect them. We like to sort our shoes by colour, but you don't have to get that fancy.

Soft shoe bags protect good shoes from scratches and bumps, and when packed in suitcases.

Store shoes where air can circulate around them. A shoe rack near the front door is a good idea in big households.

Keep shoes heeled and polished regularly to keep them looking good.

After you've worn shoes, allow them to air-dry for a few hours before putting them away in the wardrobe. Sweaty shoes can attract mildew and mould.

Suede shoes need a bit more looking after. Steam them over a kettle – don't use shampoo or cleaner – then buff up with a suede brush.

Take your outdoor shoes off when you come in the front door so you don't tread dirt and other detritus around the house. Keep your slippers there, so they're handy for when you come in.

the living environment

**APPLIANCE OF SCIENCE**
75 per cent of dust in the house is brought in on your shoes.

# Bathroom

What makes a good bathroom? We like a bath, a decent-sized shower head and good water pressure. A heated towel rail is nice too.

Who wants bottles and pots everywhere cluttering up the shelves and collecting dirt, mildew and mould? Hide away as many as you can in a cupboard with your other unmentionables. Have fresh towels and new loo rolls to hand – nothing worse than being caught short!

The bathroom is one of the muckiest rooms in the house, prone to damp, smells and mildew. Good ventilation is a must. A small vent in a ceiling or window is not enough, you'll steam the whole place up. Instead, throw open your windows and doors, and put your extractor fans on full blast. And keep the room sparkling clean. You should be able to eat your dinner off the floor!

- If you've got condensation trickling down your windows, open them wide immediately. Open doors too.

- Rinse your bath or shower cubicle out after showering. Wipe round with a soapy cloth after a bath, too.

- Get a bin with a lid for the bathroom, and empty it regularly.

- Clean and disinfect your loo pan every few days.

- Let your towels dry in the open air after using them. Hang them over a banister or drying rack rather than putting them on the radiator. Heat sets in smells.

- Towels that dry your personal bits need laundering as often as possible; wash other towels twice a week.

- Wash face flannels every day in the machine or hand wash in some biological washing powder and hang over the bath to dry.

- Wash bath mats once a week to kill off fungi and moulds.

- Wash your bathroom floor at least once a week, and immediately after an accident. Use fresh water, soap or disinfectant, and a special bathroom mop to stop cross contamination.

- If you have carpet on your bathroom floor, consider changing it for vinyl or tiles. Carpet harbours many micro-organisms and once it gets wet it's hard to keep fresh.

- Extractor fans get clogged up with dust. Take a slightly damp cloth and clean it every so often, or use the vacuum nozzle.

**STAR TIP**
When running a bath, run the amount of cold water you need first. Then fill up with hot to the right height. It prevents the bathroom steaming up so mould can't take hold.

# Watch out for your pipes

To keep your bath pipes fresh and lovely, pour down washing soda crystals and boiling water once a month. Remember to do the overflow pipe too.

Long hair clogs up sinks and baths. Ags loves to get clumps out with a plunger, or long tweezers are worth a go, too.

If you take oily baths, you'll need to take extra care. Oil collects body hair which soon bungs up pipes and drains. Every week, pour equal measures of soda crystals and salt down the plug hole. Then tip in some clear distilled vinegar with boiling water. You'll hear it sizzle as it clears out the system. But there are no miracles, so if everything is clogged up, call a plumber.

## Wash your towels twice a week. After all, they are drying all your orifices!

# Toothbrush out or toothbrush in?

Should we leave our toothbrushes out in the bathroom day and night? They can pick up airborne bacteria and odours when the loo is flushed – and then we put them straight in our mouths. Ugh, disgusting! The germs won't kill you, but why not be a bit fussy?

We'd rather be called too fussy than too slovenly any day. Putting your toothbrush away in your bathroom cabinet isn't hard. Just rinse it out, and dry on a clean towel before you put it away. Then at least you'll know it's fresh and odour free.

# For happy guests

Other people don't want to use your old soap and soggy wet hand-towels. It's like using someone else's toothbrush – who knows what kind of germs you could pick up? So please, please, please always have a pump dispenser soap in the loo when visitors come.

Nor should you put out a guest towel or, even worse, those posh bits of embroidered linen that get dripping wet after two minutes. No-one wants to use someone else's damp, soiled towels. When visitors are coming, it's nice to put out individual towels instead. Always provide an open bin so they can be dropped in and laundered later. Paper towels are another option, but never throw them down the loo as they will clog it up very quickly.

Even pump dispensers transfer germs. We don't want to get too particular, but dip your hands under the tap before you punch down the soap dispenser. Then at least you'll have put clean water between you and any nasties anybody else has deposited.

# CLEAN
# ROUTINES

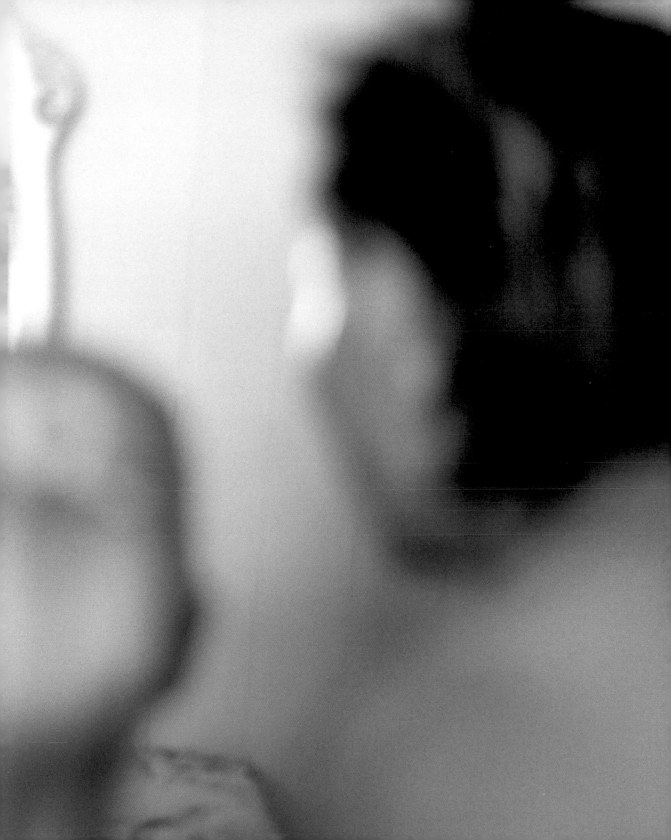

# Get into a routine

## Daily routines

To be organised is a very simple way of life. If you do the following tasks every day they will soon become second nature. A couple of minutes here, a few seconds there, and you'll soon wonder what all the fuss was about.

Put dirty clothes in the laundry basket as soon as you take them off. Fold and put away items that don't need washing, such as jeans and jumpers, before you go to bed.

Spot clean lightly soiled clothes using plain water and toilet soap on a face cloth. Then dry, air and put away.

Get into the habit of sorting through your dirty laundry every day and popping a load in the machine whenever you need to.

Air your bedding every day. Pull back the sheets while you're showering and breakfasting in the morning.

Open a window in your bedroom every day for as long as possible. It reduces humidity and will help control dust mites.

Do the rest of your household a favour – rinse out the bath after your ablutions.

# Weekly routines

It's tempting to save all of these up for a mammoth blitz at the end of the week. Don't: it always gets on top of you. Every day add one or two of these tasks to your daily routine and things will stay clean and dandy all week long.

Every few days, launder all the towels in the house on a 60°C wash.

Change and wash your bed linen once or twice a week

Change and wash your nightclothes twice a week.

Pile up used delicates separately and, once or twice a week, give them a hand-wash.

Iron the laundry. Little and often is better than one weekly blitz.

Polish leather shoes you've been wearing all week, and don't let your children go to school on a Monday with scuffed toes!

Sew on any loose buttons and repair hems where needed.

Dust around your bedroom and vacuum the floor at least once a week.

Disinfect your loo pan and wash your bathroom floor every few days. They should both be so spotless you could eat your dinner off them.

clean routines

# Monthly routines

You probably think we've gone a bit bonkers with our rigorous routines. Who'd ever do all this every month? But there's dirt you can see and there's dirt you can't. These measures attack the hidden muck that lingers beneath the surface causing allergies and irritations. Do one or two of these chores every month and you'll know your bedroom and laundry are spotless.

1 Wash your mattress and pillow protectors at 60°C.

2 Vacuum the mattress thoroughly with the crevice attachment.

3 Put your feather pillows in the freezer in a plastic bag for six hours to kill dust mites.

4 Vacuum under your bed and dust on top of wardrobes and cupboards where dust balls build up. Give the inside of the wardrobe a good going over once a month with a vacuum cleaner.

5 Wash your shower curtain to remove any spots of mildew.

6 Wash net curtains by soaking them in biological washing powder then rinsing.

7 Clean and descale the washing machine by running it empty with a cup of clear distilled vinegar.

# You probably think
## we've gone a bit bonkers…

# Spring (and autumn) cleaning

Every household used to have a big spring clean. It's not so fashionable now that electric lighting means we can see our dirt all year round! Still, it's lovely to tick off a few of these big jobs every six months.

Launder your pillows and duvet once or twice a year, and more often if you sweat a lot at night or suffer from allergies. Take them to the launderette to save your own washing machine from a pounding.

Wash or dry clean blankets, bed coverings and over-quilts at least once a year.

Change over to your summer or winter wardrobe. Before you put clothes away for the season, wash and iron them. Body oils on worn clothes attract moths and mites.

Turn your mattress once every few months to prevent dips forming.

Once a year, take down the curtains in the bedroom and either wash or dry clean them.

Vacuum or wash down the walls in your bedroom twice a year to get rid of dust and cobwebs.

Dust your bedroom lampshades with a slightly damp duster every few months.

Wash your bedroom windows. There, isn't it lovely to see out again!

# Recipes for cleanliness

## Hot date

You don't need to do much different for a big date. Of course, scrub yourself within an inch of your life beforehand – and hope he or she does too. Keep your nose out for what's happening orally, you want your breath to be sweet and fresh for that kiss moment.

Men can show they care by close shaving: shave once with the grain, then repeat against the grain for a lovely smooth finish.

Women should get the razor blade out big time, accessing all superfluous hairy areas.

Get the roll-on deodorant out before a date, and wear cotton blouses or shirts rather than synthetics to stop the ming rising.

Everyone's breath gets stale. Carry a toothbrush with you and pop to the loo for a brush-up after dinner, or use a discreet breath freshener spray.

In the first throes of romance, many a man's trigger finger gets stuck on the cologne nozzle. No woman wants a man to smell nicer than she does – we don't like the competition. Two sprays at the most or spritz some cologne into the air, then walk through it.

Never put cologne or perfume below the belt. It'll sting so much you'll be able to fry an egg on your privates.

Lipstick isn't nice to kiss. Who wants slobbery red marks all over their face? Desist, or put on just a light slick for the perfect pout.

# Job interview

Look clean. No one wants to share the office with someone who looks as if they might stink the place out. You want to appear spruce, not scary, for job interviews, so don't wear dark lips or panda eyes. This regime works well for court appearances and other official meetings, too.

Get your hair cut or put it up so it's not flapping all over your face. Always wash it that day or the day before.

Give yourself an all-over scrub, especially under your fingernails. Get your nails sorted – nothing drastic, just push back cuticles and give nails a buff up.

Pluck or trim wayward eyebrow hairs. If we were interviewing you, they'd distract us so much we wouldn't be able to listen to what you were saying.

Clean clothes, please, and no frayed edges. Press everything and get a good crease in your trousers.

Scruffy shoes are a real giveaway of a lazy beggar. Shoes don't have to be new, but they do have to be clean and not too bashed about. A bit of spit, polish and elbow grease should do the job.

If you're nervous and sweat buckets, use a 20 per cent aluminium chloride antiperspirant the night before to shut down your sweat glands (see page 99). Before you go in, put a little bicarbonate of soda on your palms to prevent a damp handshake.

Don't overdose on the aftershave or perfume. Gently spritz on a light, fresh fragrance that won't knock the interviewer for six.

Wear low-key make-up.

Have an anti-shine strategy. Before you go in, check your face isn't glowing. Place a tissue over your face, press it down and the tissue will absorb the grease, then dab on some matt powder.

Check shoulders for dandruff. Then smile, don't grimace, and in you go.

# Getting a sexy skanker to shape up

Napoleon famously liked Josephine when she smelt a little stale but clean is more of our romantic dream.

Start by explaining that you find a clean, shiny body a turn on. Give them gifts of grooming tools, shampoos, soaps and antiperspirants.

Tell him that goatees and beards are out of fashion and you find the smell of shaving cream irresistible.

Tell them you love it à deux in the shower or bath, then you can surreptitiously start lathering them.

Spill coffee over their clothes so they'll have to go home and put clean ones on.

Tell them you like to get sweaty during sex, not before it.

Jump out of bed saying that something has bitten you. Insist on clean sheets, or you're leaving.

Go on a sex strike. It worked for Lysistrata, it could work for you. If all else fails, dump them. But do us all a favour and tell them why.

# So you're going travelling . . .

For some of you mucky pups, staying clean is a challenge at home, never mind when you're staying in grotty, foreign rooms with bed bugs, lice and no running water. Make it simple by taking easy-care clothes, stacks of toilet soap and washing your hands every chance you get.

**Before you go**

◯ Cut your hair short. It makes it easier to care for and head lice infestations less likely.

◯ Travel light, taking only a few clothes that are wash and wear.

◯ Leave your powder puffs and aftershave at home and take an antiperspirant, heavy-duty sunscreen, soap, medicines and feet care treatments instead. Ask your pharmacist for advice.

**While you're there**

◯ You can wash your whole body with a face flannel and a small bowl of cold water (see page 44). Then wash out the face flannel with toilet soap and leave to dry.

◯ Wash clothes with toilet soap, but don't put too much on. When water is in short supply it's difficult to rinse properly and the residue can cause skin rashes.

◯ Take a pack of antiseptic wipes for emergency handwashing when no water is available. Cut them in half so they last longer.

**When you get back**

◯ Jump in a hot bath and scrub your body all over with antibacterial soap. Wash hair under a shower. Let all the water out and re-run it. Then do the same again.

◯ If hair is fibrillating with head lice, cut it short, wash well, buy a nit lotion from a pharmacist, then delouse yourself with a nit comb. Repeat every few days until all live lice and nit eggs are out.

# So you're a smoker…

You can't smell good if you're a smoker. Masking the smell of smoke with perfumes and air fresheners doesn't work – it's just wallpapering over the cracks. Our number one tip is to stop smoking, you stinkers, but failing that:

1 Shower and wash your hair every day. Using a soap with a herby fragrance such as rosemary can help counteract the niff.

2 If hair is long, think about getting it cut shorter. Long hair smells sour if exposed to smoke. Try rubbing some dried lavender into hair then brushing it out. Bicarbonate of soda can work as a dry shampoo.

3 Brush teeth three times a day. Brush or scrape your tongue, too. Smokers and drinkers are more susceptible to the oral bacteria which cause bad breath.

4 Think about a mouthwash. Use one without alcohol, which can dry out the mouth more.

5 Chew parsley or cloves throughout the day to freshen up the oral pong.

6 When you come back from the pub, put clothes on a hanger and stick them out the back door or on a balcony at night to air. If you don't have outside space, hang them in the bathroom, where the steam will help extract the smoky ming.

7 Don't smoke in the house and especially not in the bedroom. All your soft furnishings will collect the smell and it will linger for ever.

8 Last but not least, be considerate to non-smokers.

# So you get dirty every day …

Artists, builders, dustmen and farmers get filthy every day. Wear protective clothing, especially gloves, whenever you can.

Before going to work, use a nailbrush to apply a layer of soap beneath your nails. It stops filth and germs from gathering there.

Rub a little handcream into hands – not so much that they become slippery – before you start work. It makes it easier to get the dirt off later.

To clean under short nails, use an orange stick (available at any pharmacy) or a nailbrush.

Farmers are at risk of getting highly toxic *E. Coli 0157* bacteria on their hands from animal faeces. Wash hands very regularly and avoid touching your mouth and nose.

Cover cuts immediately with plasters, and keep chafed skin moisturised so it stays infection free.

After the day's work always shower, or bathe, and wash hair as soon as you get home.

index

# Index

acne 37, 61, 101, 102–5
aftershave 83
allergies 20, 35, 77, 143
almond oil 125
aluminium chloride 99, 114, 185
ammonium alum crystal 99
antiperspirants 99
    stains 152
apple cider vinegar 49
aqueous cream 62
athlete's foot 57, 112
avocado 78

bacteria 36–7
bad breath 75, 89, 90, 188
    fresheners 94
baking soda 91, 99
banana facial 62
bath mitt 49
bathrooms 174–7
baths/bathing 23, 27, 48–9
beards 85
bed bugs 33
bed covers 169
bedrooms 162–71
beer 78
bicarbonate of soda 118, 135, 168
blackheads 105
blood stains 152
body piercings 156
body scrubber/scrubs 45, 49
bras 142–3, 144
breath fresheners 94
butter stains 153

candlewax stains 152
chewing gum stains 152
chocolate stains 152
cleaning routines 180–3
clothes care 172
clothes hangers 172
clothes washing see washing
    clothes
coffee stains 152
cold sores 107
conditioner, hair 24, 29, 78
conjunctivitis 106

contact lens care 96
cornflour 118
cucumber facial 62

dandruff 80
dating 184
dental floss 24, 27, 92
denture cleaning tablets 153
dentures, cleaning 91
deodorants 24, 29, 99
    stains 152
dreadlocks 79
dry-cleaning 145
dry skin 61, 62
drying clothes 146–7
dust mites 20, 77, 143, 163, 164
dust/dusting 162, 163
duvets 169

ears 97
E.coli 37, 55, 189
egg facial 62
emery boards 27, 121
Epsom salts 49, 115
exfoliation 45, 49, 62, 71
eyebrows 107
eyes 96

face
    skin types 61
    washing 44, 58–62
facials 62
feet 110–19
    cracked heels 26
    deodorisers 115
    diseases 112–13
    home pedicure 119
    moisturising of 71
    rough skin healer 115
    smelly 75, 114
    stinky shoe and sock care 118
    sweaty 57, 114
    treatments 115
    washing 56–7
five-minute boil wash 44
flannels, face 27, 47
food poisoning 37, 52

foundation 106
fungi 35
gardening hand scrub 125
ginger 49
gold jewellery 156
grass stains 153
grease stains 153
grey hair 78, 80
grooming essentials 22–9
gum disease 90
gym gear 156

hair 77–81
    brightening dull 79
    camouflaging grey 78
    conditioning 24, 29, 78
    and dandruff 80
    dreadlocks 79
    enhancing colour of 78
    getting rid of split ends 79
    managing curly 78
    shine on dry 78
    treatments for 78–9
    washing 44, 77
hairbrush 23, 26, 81
hand cream 29, 53, 69, 125, 189
hands 120–7
    cure for dry and scaly 125
    illnesses spread by dirty 41,
        50, 52
    removing stains 125
    sweaty palms cure 125
    washing 50–3
    see also nails
head lice 35, 77, 187
hyperhidrosis 114

impetigo 84
ink stains 153
iontophoresis 114
ironing 149–50
itchiness, ways to stop 49

jewellery 156
job interview 185

ketchup stains 153

laundry *see* washing clothes
laundry baskets 135
lemon foot wash 115
lemons 49, 94, 125
lice
    body 35
    head 35, 77, 187
lipstick stains 153
*Listeria* 37

make-up 106
    stains 153
mascara 106
mattresses 168
mayonnaise 78
*Microbial keratitis* 96
mildew stains 153
milk bath 49
moisturising skin 29, 49, 61
mud stains 153
myrrh 62

nails 120–7
    biting 127
    cleaning under 26, 189
    cure for brittle and split 125
    enriching 125
    false 126
    filing 27, 121
    germs and bacteria 50, 120
    home manicure 122–3
    keeping strong 127
    removing stains from 125
nappies, washing 155

oat facial wash 62
oatmeal body scrub 45
oil stains 153
oily skin 61

peach facial 62
perspiration stains 153
pierced ears 97
pillows/pillowcases 164
pitted keratolysis 113
poison ivy 107
*Propionibacterium acnes*
    37
*Pseudomonas* 37
public loos 55
pumice stone 26, 57

razors 22, 27, 84
rings, cleaning under 156
rosewater 61
    and vodka aftershave 83
rubber gloves 122

sage
  and pine foot fresheners 115
  rinse 78
*Salmonella* 37
scabies 34
*Serratia* 37, 96
shampoo 24, 29
shaving 83–7, 184
    aftershave 83
    electric shaving routine 85
    of head 86
    legs 87
    nicking yourself 83
    underarms 86
    wet blade care 84
    wet shaving routine 84
sheets
    getting white 139
    ironing cotton 150
    washing 166
shoes 118, 119, 173, 185
silk, washing 140
silver jewellery 156
skin
    brushing 69
    exfoliating 45, 49, 62, 71
    invigorating and stimulating
      circulation 49
    moisturising 29, 49, 61
    types of 61
smoking 188
soap 24, 29, 63
socks 118, 136
splinters 107
split ends 79
spot cleaning 145
spots 37, 60 *see also* acne
stains
    removing from clothes 151–3
    removing from hands/nails 125
*Staphylococcus aureus* 37, 84, 156
sunburn, relief for 107
sweat glands 42, 57, 75
sweating 41, 42, 99
swimmer's ear 97

tea 115
tea stains 152
tea tree oil 57, 105, 118
teeth 90–4
    brushing 90, 92
    cleaning of dentures 91
    whitening 91
tomato stains 153
tongue brushing 90, 92
toothbrushes 22, 26, 92, 177
toothpaste 24, 29, 91
torso sluice 46
towels 23, 27, 175
travelling 137, 187
tumble dryers 147
tummy button 75

underarms 98–9
    shaving 86
    *see also* deodorants
underwear 141–3, 172

vegetable shortening
    115, 125
vinegar 78
vitamin E 105

wardrobe 171, 172
washing
    reasons for 41
    routines 68–9
washing clothes 130–45
    allergy prevention 143
    bleeding into rest of wash
      134, 144
    by hand 137
    by machine 136, 144
    dry-cleaning 145
    pilling and bobbling 144
    powders and detergents 31
    silk 140
    sorting the laundry 134,
      144
    stain removing 151–3
    temperature control 132
    traveller's tricks 137
    underwear 141–3
    whiter and brighter 138–9
watches 156
wine stains 152
witch hazel 62

# Acknowledgements

Many thanks to:

Jane Philimore, the writer; Steph Harris who developed the idea, produced the pilot and edited the series; Lyn Rowett, the series producer; Derren Ready, our microbiologist; Ben Frow who came up with the title and oversaw the pilot; Sue Murphy, the commissioning editor who oversaw the series.

The Penguin team: Kate Adams, Abbie and Jane in publicity, Gillian Haslam, all at Smith & Gilmour, photographer Mark Read and his assistant Darren and Cat Ledger.

K-West Hotel and Spa for allowing us to take photos there.

The soap-dodgers: Amy, Osla, Joseph, Barry, Dan, Richie and Stefan.

The team who worked on the series: Will Cross, Andrew Nelson, Kate Moray, Claire Hobday, Will Hicklin, Danny Fildes, Lesley Brandon, Jenny Freilich, Katie Atwood, Gordon Maxwell, Jon Durbridge, Rob Rawlins, Charlotte Bridger, Hugo and Vicky and Huge, Magpie, Fusion, Mike Hayley, Al Collingwood, Gemma Shanley, Rob, David, Raquel and Francis.

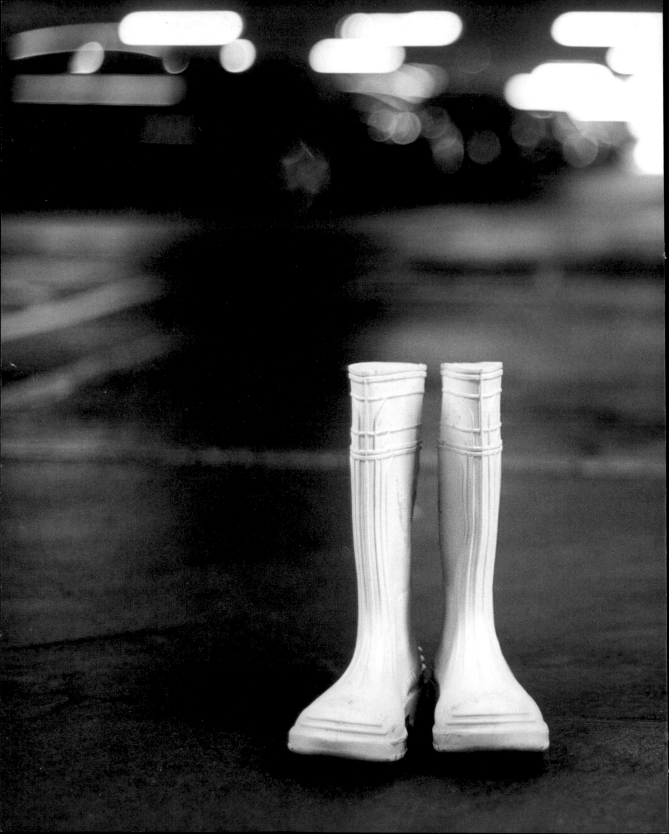